Careers in Medicine for the New Woman

Careers in Medicine for the New Woman

by Carol Jochnowitz

CHOOSING CAREERS AND LIFE-STYLES

Franklin Watts/New York/London/1978

Photographs by Steven Rudley

Library of Congress Cataloging in Publication Data

Jochnowitz, Carol.
Careers in medicine for the new woman.

(Choosing careers and life-styles)
Includes index.
SUMMARY: Discusses the qualities needed to become a physician, medical schools, training, and specialities within medicine. Also includes brief interviews with women in medicine.
1. Women physicians—Juvenile literature. 2. Medicine—Vocational guidance—Juvenile literature. 3. Nursing—Vocational guidance—Juvenile literature. [1. Women physicians. 2. Medicine—Vocational guidance. 3. Nursing—Vocational guidance. 4. Vocational guidance] I. Title.
R692.J6 610.69 77-17226
ISBN 0-531-01444-4

Printed in the United States of America
5 4 3 2 1

This book is dedicated to the memory of my father
George Fink

Contents

Careers in Medicine for the New Woman

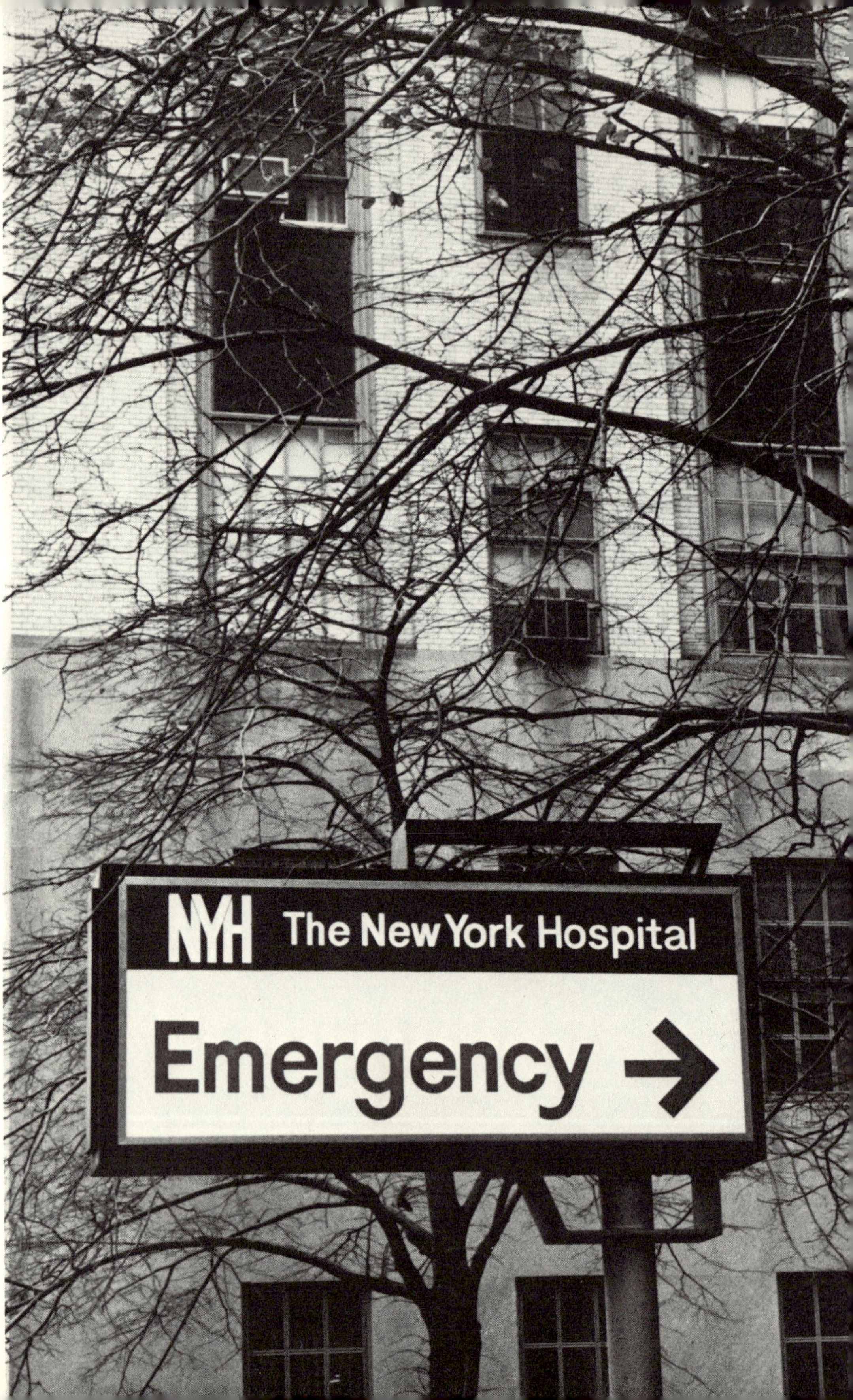
NYH The New York Hospital
Emergency

1

Introduction

> A man and his son are driving along a highway at night when their car suddenly goes out of control and smashes into a truck. The father is killed instantly; the son is rushed to the nearest hospital, in critical condition and in need of immediate surgery. He is put on the operating table. The surgeon steps up, looks at him, and falls back, gasping, "I can't do it—I can't operate on this boy! He's my own son!"
>
> How is this possible?

When this riddle made the rounds a few years ago, most people could not figure it out. Ask it a few years from now, however, and chances are the people you question will have much less difficulty coming up with the answer. The record should help us understand why.

In 1905, women made up 4 percent of all U.S. medical school graduates. Sixty years later, that number had risen to only 7.3 percent. By 1972, it was 9 percent. But, in 1971, the number of women *entering* American medical schools was 13.5 percent of total enrollment. By 1972, that number had risen to 16.8 percent. In 1974 it was 22.3 percent; in 1976, 24.7 per-

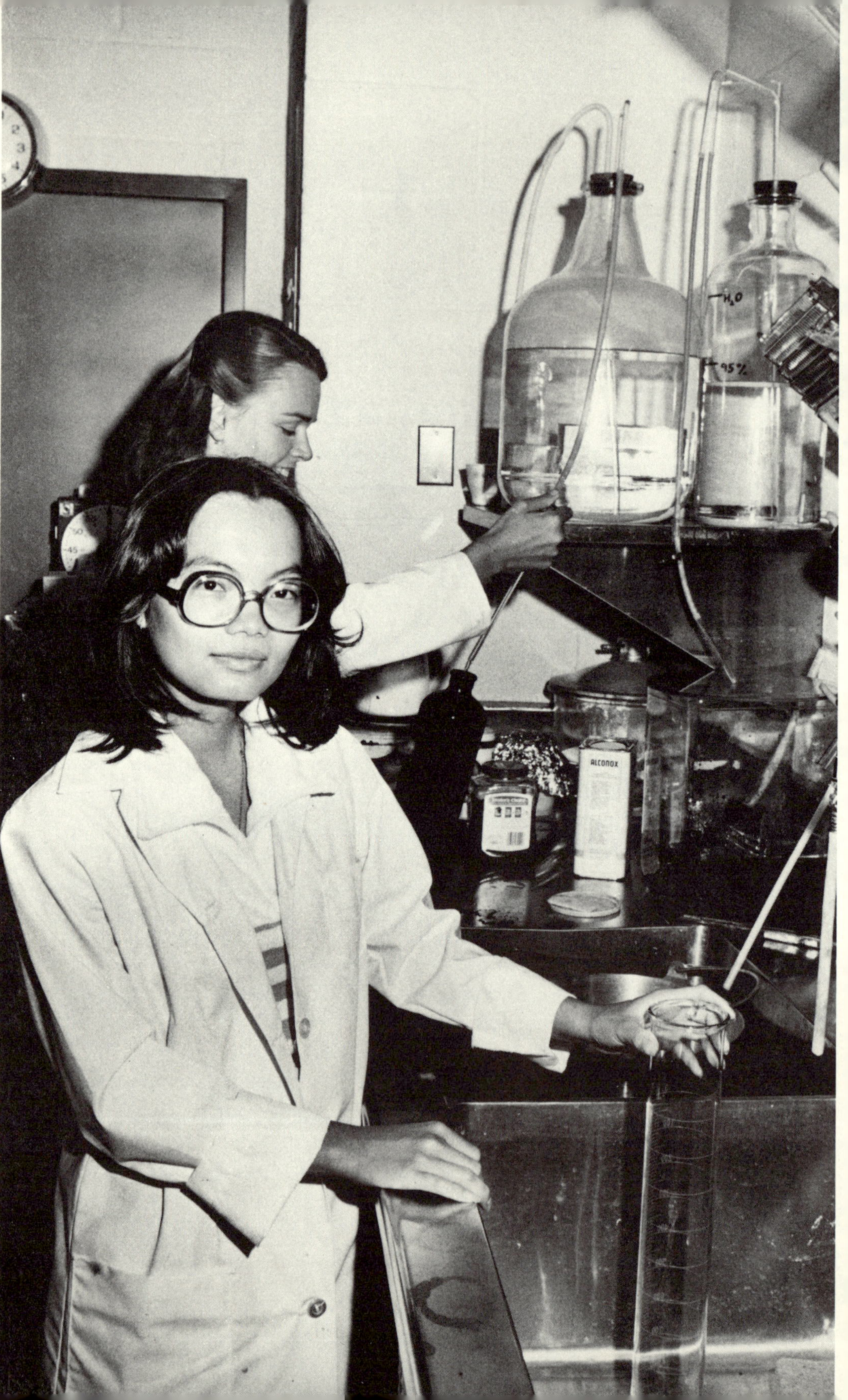
H2O
95%
ALCONOX

cent! In most European countries women make up 20–30 percent of the medical profession, and at least three-quarters of all doctors in the Soviet Union are women. As of 1970, women accounted for only 7–8 percent of all the physicians in the U.S. By 1980, however, their number should have risen to one-quarter or more of all the people entering the medical profession in this country each year. Some medical schools, such as the one at the State University of New York at Stonybrook, already have classes which are almost 50 percent female.

Although the increase in women medical students in the early 1970's was dramatic, it was not the result of a sudden decision on the part of the medical schools to admit women en masse. As Carol Lopate pointed out in her book, *Women in Medicine,* the number of women admitted to medical schools each year has always been a reflection of the number applying. The increased number of women entering medicine is due instead to the changing attitude of today's woman about the kind of life she wants.

Not only has the attitude of women changed. The medical profession itself was not always ready to welcome women. In the nineteenth century, the idea of a woman in medicine or in any other profession outside of schoolteaching was unthinkable to most people. When Elizabeth Blackwell graduated from Geneva Medical College in 1849, thus becoming the first woman in the United States to receive a medical degree, she was initiating a struggle against popular opinion and establishment opposition that was to continue for more than fifty years. The American Medical Women's Association, founded in 1915 (the

The last few years have seen a dramatic increase in the number of women who have decided to enter medicine. This young doctor works at an eye institute. Her research may lead to a more effective treatment for cataracts.

same year the American Medical Association decided to admit women to membership), has had to devote much of its time and effort to the fight for equal rights for women in the medical profession. As it is, however, it has a long history of progressive positions on such issues as birth control, abortion, and medical insurance.

The women who went to medical school a generation or two ago were not regarded as unnatural creatures, as were their nineteenth-century predecessors, but they weren't emancipated, either. "My generation thought we were being *allowed* to go to medical school. We thought we had to be good little girls," one woman recalled. Another said, "I took it for granted that there would be prejudice, and there was. I had a much higher tolerance for frustration than the young women I see today. They won't put up with inferior facilities or snide remarks any more. We never complained; we felt lucky just to be there."

It is true that young women today do not regard the opportunity to study medicine as any kind of special privilege. Most would probably agree with the woman who said, "I've always thought of myself as a doctor, not as a 'woman' doctor." When they do encounter the occasional professor who does not like women who smoke and/or wear pants, or the male colleague who just doesn't believe that a woman could ever be as good a doctor as a man, they tend to regard those attitudes as the problem of those who hold them. Such prejudices are certainly not something that would affect the commitment to study and practice medicine. "Of course there are going to be people who are prejudiced against women," they say. "Of course you're going to meet patients who don't want a woman doctor. That doesn't matter. You just stand your ground, put in your time, do what you have to do, and they will see that you are capable and determined."

What makes a woman decide to become a doctor, and what is she like? Some women say that they had known they wanted to become doctors from the time they were four or five years old. One remembered: "My uncle started medical school when

I started first grade, and I always knew I would do the same thing. I knew I was smart and could do anything I wanted." Having a physician in the family can help to direct a young girl's ambition, but what is more important is that her parents give her confidence in herself. "When you open that office door for the first time, not knowing where your first patient is coming from—that's the moment of truth," one physician said. "Your parents have to have convinced you that you're great." Some women remember having a parent—usually the father—counsel them that a woman should always have a profession that eventually could make her financially independent.

Other women report that they were moved to study medicine by the death or illness of someone they loved. They responded to their personal tragedies by resolving to do something to alleviate human suffering. One doctor made her decision at the age of fifteen, when a neighbor was overcome by carbon monoxide and she was able to save his life because of training in a first-aid course she had taken. "He looked on me as his savior," she recalled. "I liked the idea of being a savior."

For most women, however, the decision to enter the medical profession does not result from a single incident, but instead comes from a slowly gathering conviction throughout adolescence that this is the work they want to do. Most will say that it is impossible to pinpoint exactly when they decided. Typical comments are: "I was always interested in science, and it just evolved," or, "I knew I wanted to do something with science, but in such a way that I would be helping people directly."

The desire to serve humanity has always ranked high among the reasons given for going into medicine, and, in fact, one would not be worth much as a doctor without it. That alone, however, is not sufficient. You *must* have the talent for and an interest in science as well. It is extremely difficult to get into medical school, and you must have superior grades in science all through college in order to be admitted. Once you are admitted, you will find yourself embarked on four years of the most rigorous, vigorous, and demanding education required by any profession. In fact, some professors have expressed concern at how completely medical training tends to take over students' minds. They worry in particular about female students, whose higher dropout rate, some think, may be due to the fact that women have not been socially conditioned to have the steely determination and personal assertiveness needed to meet the pressure.

Once training is behind you, however, what is it like being a doctor? One medical school admissions officer said that a major part of the practice of medicine consisted of solving problems. It may be that remembering one little fact will finally make sense out of an assortment of symptoms and allow a diagnosis to fall into place. One doctor recalled a woman who kept returning to a clinic with the same complaint—swollen glands. There was no apparent cause for the condition, and everyone thought it must be cancer. The woman was diabetic and the doctor recalled something she had read years before—that in a patient with diabetes, certain infections prove uniquely resistant to the patient's own antibodies. Antibiotics were prescribed and the swelling went away. "All my life I've been accused of acting on hunches," she said. "Now I know they're educated hunches and I won't back down."

Another doctor had this to say to a woman considering medicine: "Be sure you can take it." Doctors are exposed to sights that most people are mercifully spared. It's a part of their commitment. But most say that, thanks to constant exposure, you get over many of your adverse reactions by your second year of medical school.

This pediatric endocrinologist's job responsibilities include counseling for diabetics. Her patients depend upon her professional expertise to keep them alive.

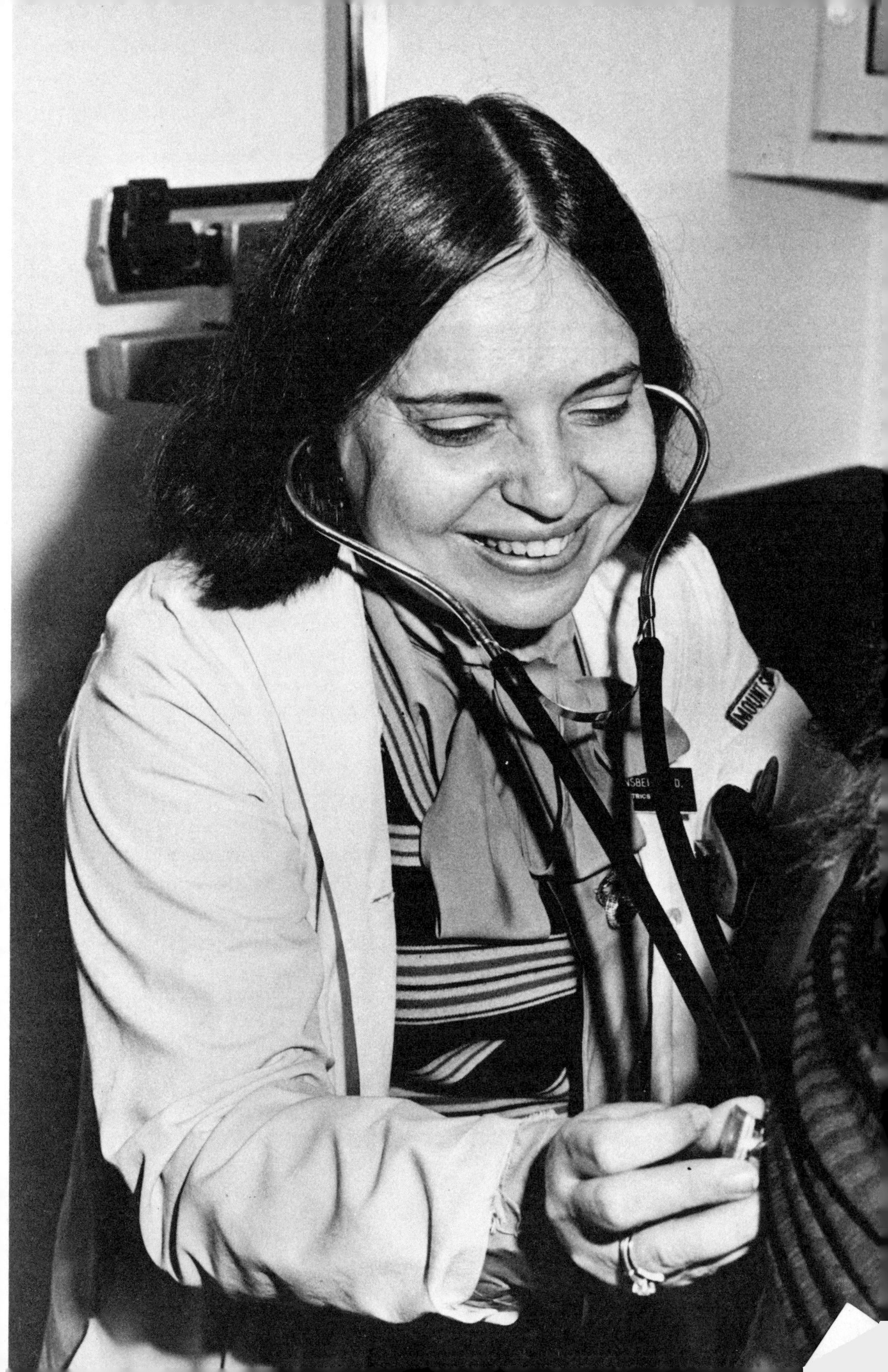

Doctors also see patients die—adults and children alike. They see people who are terrified, people overwhelmed with grief. A good doctor is never inured to such things. She does not say, as she will of the unpleasant things uncovered in her anatomy and pathology courses, "After a while it doesn't bother you any more." But she keeps herself strong enough to be strong for other people. Doctors are often the only people present at the most terrifying moments of human life, and people expect their training and experience to have given them all the answers. Many people believe women are better at these junctures than are men, more able to empathize, less apt to appear unfeeling—whether because of an innate personality difference, as some people believe, or because our society allows women to be more open about their emotions.

The first thing most doctors have to say about medicine is how much they love it. "I consider it a calling," one said. "Some people think it's overly sentimental to use words like that. I don't agree."

"One of the real joys is the feeling of being on a team," one woman said. "From the head of the department down through the interns, the nurses, the aides, even the elevator operators! You're sharing human life. When you're doing something like that as your life's work, it makes it worthwhile to get up in the morning."

"My husband and I went to Guatemala to work in a tiny hospital on top of a mountain so high even the mules couldn't make it all the way up," said another. "We couldn't even speak the language, but we could do enough so that every Sunday the priest thanked God for sending us. If you practice it properly and appropriately, it's a tremendous gift. If you feel put upon, if you don't like to give—then it's not for you. I would never try to *persuade* anyone to be a doctor—there's a very long gestation period—but if you *can* be one, I can't imagine why you'd ever want to be anything else."

2

The Way to Medical School

It is possible that you could be on the way to medical school now. A few colleges, in conjunction with affiliated medical schools, offer six-year programs which award both a Bachelor of Science degree and an M.D. In other words, if you apply successfully to such a program, you are admitted to both college and medical school at the same time. Some of these programs compress the work for each four-year degree into three years; some begin the medical curriculum after two years, with the remaining undergraduate work to be completed during summer sessions; some use the classroom requirements for the medical degree in place of the various college electives. Among the schools currently offering such programs are Boston University, Brown University, the University of Michigan, the City College of New York, Pennsylvania State University, and the University of Missouri.

If you apply successfully to one of these programs, you will not only have given yourself a two-year headstart on your medical career, but you will also have taken care of college and med-school admissions at the same time. And applying to medical school, as you will learn later, is a long and complicated business, routinely causing thousands of pre-medical seniors months of anxiety each year. Still, there are disadvantages to such programs too. Most of them require full-time course loads throughout at least some of the summers, and six years is a long time to go to school without a break. Also, you are propelled into a career two years ahead of time. As one doctor who had been through such a course remarked, "It means that in medical school you're two years younger than anybody else, and I don't know if that's such a good thing. You're less mature at a time in your life when you need a lot of maturity." In addition, it is worth noting that there was a 50 percent dropout rate in the accelerated course this particular doctor was in, whereas the average attrition rate in medical school is no more than 15 percent for women (8 percent for men). The college experience, after all, does a great deal to shape a person's character and plans, and sometimes it may change her mind entirely. (In the case of pre-med students, a course in organic chemistry is particularly famous for altering career plans.)

So the six-year option is something you should not rush into unless you are exceptionally sure of your ambition and aptitude for a career in medicine. Ask yourself some questions: Is it something you would want to work at for the rest of your life? Are you more interested in science than most students? Are your grades in science courses consistently high? Do you find that the more complicated something gets, the more you want to pursue it? Are you a good student generally? Do you enjoy studying just for the sake of studying? If you want to commit yourself to medical training while you are still in high school, you have to be sure that you are not only "college material," but that you are something more besides. It calls for tremendous dedication.

If, on the other hand, like most students planning a medical career, you intend to take college and medical school one at a time, the following is a description of what you will have to do as an undergraduate. Most medical schools have approximately the same subject requirements—one year each of physics, biology or zoology, and organic and inorganic chemistry, with additional work in such areas as calculus, physical chemistry, and genetics or embryology recommended. *There is no such subject or major as "pre-med,"* even if most students planning to go to medical school do give that as their answer when asked their major. And, although most pre-med students do major in science, it is not required.

The best person to see about all this is your school's or college's pre-med advisor. He or she is a faculty member designated to provide the kind of information that pre-med students need—what schools are best for each person, what the exact requirements are for each, and so forth. You can also send away for an extremely helpful booklet, *Medical School Requirements: USA and Canada,* which is published by the Association of American Medical Colleges (AAMC). It provides an alphabetical listing of all the accredited medical schools in the United States and Canada, giving their admissions requirements, the factors they consider in selecting their students, information about tuition, and so forth. You can get it by sending $5.00 ($6.50 if you want it by airmail) to AAMC, Attention: Membership and Subscriptions, One Dupont Circle, Washington, D.C., 20036. It is a good idea to send away for this booklet early in your studies, when you will still have the maximum amount of time available to decide on the best program for you. You might also want to have another booklet, available from the same source and for the same price, called the *AAMC Curriculum Directory,* which lists the curriculum and matriculation requirements for every North American medical school.

Once you have studied these materials and talked with your advisor, you should be able to decide to which schools you want to apply. It is a good idea to make this decision before the spring of your junior year in college, because that is probably when you will be taking the Medical College Admissions Test (MCAT), and you will have to indicate at that time which schools you want to receive your test scores.

The MCAT is administered twice a year, in May and September, at colleges all over the country. You can get a registration blank for it, along with an information booklet listing test centers, sample questions, and other useful things, by writing to MCAT Registration, The American College Testing Program, P.O. Box 414, Iowa City, Iowa, 52240.

The MCAT is administered in three segments: science, which in turn is divided into sections on biology, physics, and chemistry; quantitative ability (math); and verbal ability. Like the SAT students must take before entering college, the MCAT is not really a test for which you can study, and the AAMC neither sponsors nor recommends any of the "cram" aids currently on the market. Actually, most medical school admissions officers report that they give test results somewhat less weight in making their decisions than they do the three other factors—college grades, references, and the personal interview. It is true that they would conclude from a very low set of scores that you probably could not make it through medical school, but what they are really looking for is very good grades in college, especially in science courses. On the other hand, if your grades in school are very good, and your MCAT scores are low, the admissions office may conclude that your college gave "inflated" grades (an increasingly common complaint among academicians these days) and discount them accordingly.

As noted previously, your letters of recommendation are also very important. Unlike people going on to other areas of graduate study, you will not be able to select all references yourself. The medical schools want at least one to be written by an impartial third party, namely your college's own pre-med committee, which will interview you and review your grades for that purpose. The committee will be impartial when it writes its report, if for no other reason than to keep its college's credibility in good repair with the medical schools for the generations of applicants yet to come.

Finally, sometime before late autumn of your senior year you will file your applications and see to it that your college sends transcripts of your grades to all the schools you have chosen. When you went to college you probably did not apply to more than five or ten places; now you will be applying to ten or fifteen.

Medical schools do, indeed, have very high admissions requirements. At the best schools the number of students admitted may be as low as 8 percent of all who apply. Of course, the volume of applications received is partly the result of the large number of applications each individual sends out. And the difficulty students have in gaining admission is partly the result of the fact that we would need probably *twice* the number of medical schools we presently have in this country in order to accommodate *all* of the qualified applicants. You may have your sights set on one of the best schools in the country—Johns Hopkins, for example, or Stanford, or Columbia—and if you want to go there, then by all means apply. Just be sure in addition to include a number of less well-known schools.

The AAMC has set up a national clearing house, the American Medical College Application Service (AMCAS), which can simplify things if you are applying to any of the 80-odd schools registered with it. Instead of sending individual applications to each of these schools, you simply fill out a master form made up by AMCAS, which will then send it—along with your MCAT scores and college grades—to whatever schools you indicate. A list of all AMCAS schools comes with the form, which you can get by writing to AMCAS, 1776 Massachusetts Ave. NW, Suite 301, Washington, D.C., 20036. There is a fee of $10 if you want one application sent out, $15 for two, $20 for three, and so on. For most applicants, the chief beauty of this system is not so much the amount of repetitive paperwork they are spared as is the fact that they have to write only *one* essay for all their AMCAS applications. (All medical school applications require you to answer at least one essay question about your interest in and commitment to medicine, and for most applicants this is psychologically the most demanding part of the whole process.) Also, the AMCAS system may save you money. Medical schools require an application fee, ranging generally from $20 to $30, and if you are sending out even as few as ten applications, it can run into quite a sum. Your AMCAS schools, however, will demand these fees only if they pass favorably on your application and decide to call you for an interview.

With all these advantages, however, you still should not expect to be able to handle your applications exclusively through AMCAS, since there are a great many medical schools in the country which do not use it, including such places as Harvard, Yale, and Johns Hopkins. Most state university medical schools are registered with AMCAS, however, and it certainly should be of some use to you.

While you have been taking care of all these details, your medical school has not been idle. Its admissions office is awash in applications—at most institutions as many as four or five thousand students will apply each year. Of these, no more than a third will be selected to come for interviews.

One dean of admissions described the medical school interview as an attempt to measure four things: general intelligence, preparedness (how much math and science do you know?), motivation, and aptitude (do you like people, and do you enjoy solving difficult, complex problems?). You may also be asked if you have had any experience in research or patient-related work; if you have, it may be to your advantage.

It is possible—although not inevitable—that you will be asked if you are engaged to be married, and, if so, whether you intend to get pregnant at any point during your training. One outstanding pre-med student, practically assured of admission to a school that is considered particularly difficult for women to get into, was given a lecture by the interviewer on the necessity of avoiding pregnancy during the years of training. It made the student so angry she withdrew her application. What your own attitude will be with regard to this matter is something you will have to decide for yourself.

Your interviewer will write up a report which will be submitted to the school's admissions committee. You should receive notification of their decision some time before June. There is some encouragement in the fact that statistics are on your side—the proportion of female applicants who are accepted for admission each year is slightly higher than for males.

What if, in spite of the number of schools you applied to, you did not get accepted by any, but still don't want to give up the idea of being a doctor? There is something you can do. Each year a number of American pre-med students go to medical schools in foreign countries. Generally speaking, they are easier to get into and will often take students who could not find a place in any medical school here. The schools at the Universities of Bologna and Milan, in Italy, and at Guadalajara in Mexico, are among the most popular for this purpose. Think very carefully before you avail yourself of this option, however. While some European medical schools, notably those of Great Britain, Germany, and the Scandinavian countries, are excellent, many others are far inferior to their American counterparts. Instead of the small classes and tutorials which characterize American medical training, these foreign schools have to make do with enormous lecture halls. And there is practically none of the intensive, on-the-ward patient contact which any American student encounters as a matter of course from the beginning. In these foreign schools it is almost all done by the book. The result is that foreign medical graduates are almost totally unequipped to cope with the rigors of an American internship. In fact, the AMA's Council on Medical Education found it necessary in 1957 to set up a special body, the Educational Council for Foreign Medical Graduates (ECFMG), to deal with this problem. The Council administers a special qualifying exam, given twice a year, which foreign medical graduates must be able to pass. In addition, there are special requirements which these graduates must meet before they can go on to a residency in an American hospital. For American students who go to a foreign school, the ECFMG has set up something called the "Fifth Pathway," which offers the student a chance to take a junior internship or clinical clerkship for a year at a domestic school especially approved for the purpose. This enables the student to omit a regular internship, but she must take the certifying exam and submit her academic record for review. If you want very badly to become a doctor, and you find that the only way you can do it is by going to a foreign medical school, then you should probably go ahead. But be aware that you will be putting yourself at a considerable disadvantage once you get back home.

One final thing remains to be discussed with regard to admission to medical school, and that is money. As of this writing, a good private school costs about $6000 a year—and state-supported schools only charge about a thousand dollars less. Very few people can meet such costs out of their own pockets. "The rational thing to do," said one admissions officer with a touch of exasperation, "would be to abolish tuition, get the necessary money entirely from public revenue, and have the student pay it back in the form of service in an undersupplied area after graduation." Some legislators, Senator Edward M. Kennedy among them, agree. For the present, however, most students must try to get grants and loans.

Some loans are available from the schools themselves—they decide the amount you need based on a confidential statement from your parents as to their financial capabilities. Other loans come from various public and private sources. The AMA has published a Financial Information National Directory (FIND) which lists over 1,500 sources for loans, grants, and scholarships to students in health and allied professions, categorized by state and specialty. The Directory costs $2.95, and you can get it by writing to AMA, 535 North Dearborn Street, Chicago, Ill., 60610. In addition, the AMA Education and Research Foundation runs a national program guaranteeing low-interest bank loans for students, interns, and residents, to be repaid after their training is completed. A similar program for loans, offered to women students on the basis of need, is run by the American Medical Women's Association, 1740 Broadway, New York, N.Y., 10019. You might also get some useful information by writing to the Graduate and Professional School Financial Aid Service (GAPSFAS), Box 2614, Princeton, N.J., 08540, and the American Association of University Women, 2401 Virginia Avenue NW, Washington, D.C., 20037.

As for scholarships, most schools can no longer afford to offer many of them, although you should ask your pre-med advisor about their availability at the schools you would like to attend. Harvard, for example, once proclaimed that it would guarantee the tuition of any student who was outstanding enough to be admitted. This is no longer the case—Harvard now tries to make sure of having summer jobs or some other source of income available for needy students.

Two additional sources of scholarships are the Armed Forces and the United States Public Health Service (USPHS). The Armed Forces will pay your tuition, supply money for books and fees, and add a monthly stipend. In return, they require four years of service when you graduate. The USPHS makes the same stipulation. It does not provide any money for books and fees, but its stipend is considerably larger than that given by the Armed Forces.

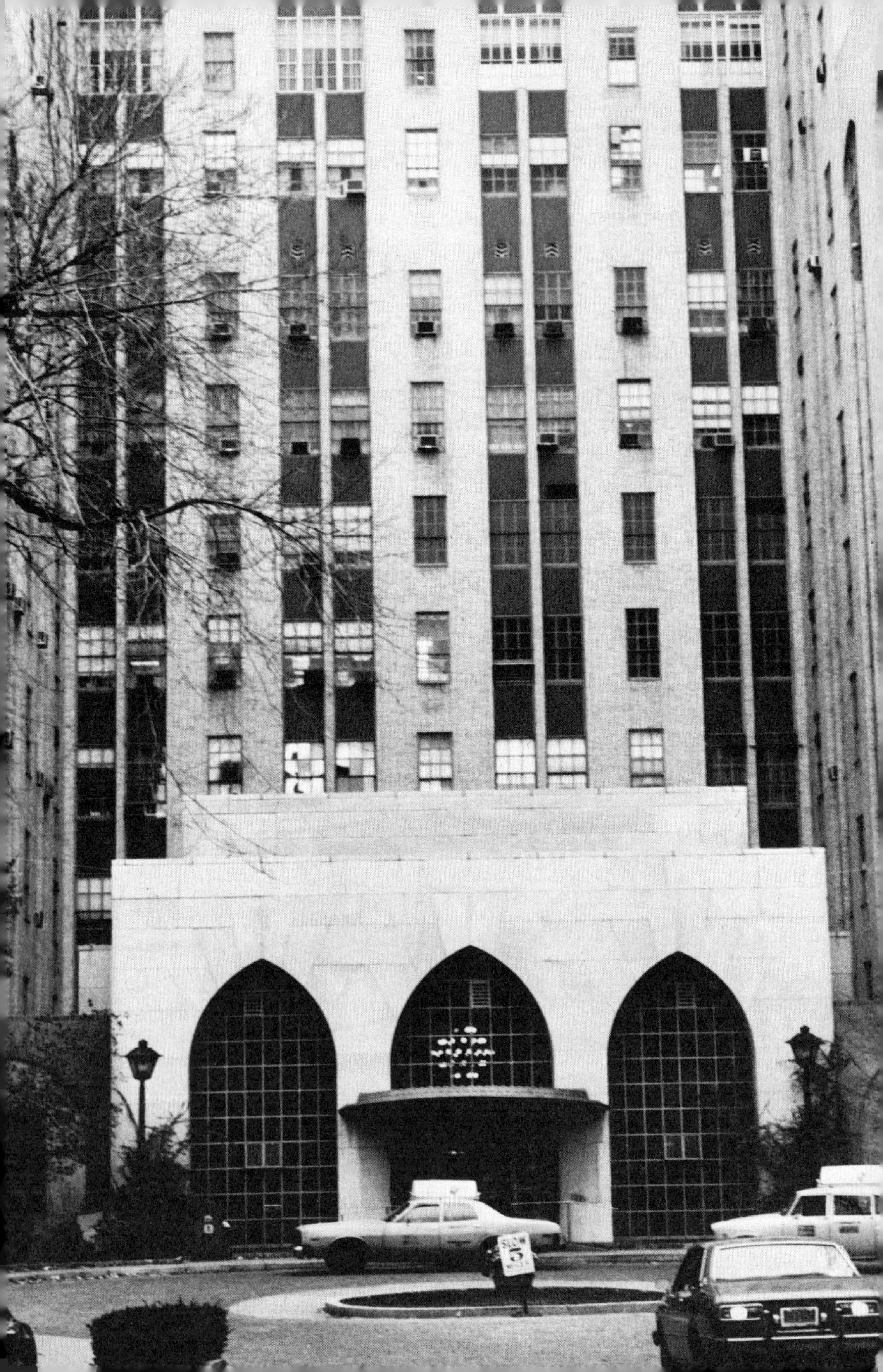
SLOW
5

3

Medical Training

The training for a medical career is divided into three parts. First, you will attend medical school for four years. In the course of these four years you will take Parts I and II of the National Board Exams, which you will almost certainly pass if you are getting passing marks in medical school. Then you will graduate, take the Oath of Hippocrates (if your school administers it), and be a doctor.

But you cannot practice yet. Before you can do that, you will have to be licensed by the state in which you will be working, and for that you must work one year as an intern and pass either Part III of the National Boards or the special state licensing exam (FLEX). Most states allow graduates of American medical schools to take the National Boards for licensure and only require the FLEX of foreign medical graduates.

An internship is a year of intensive hospital work. You apply for your internship during the last year of medical school. Application is made through the National Intern and Resident Matching Program (NIRMP), and works as follows: You will make a list of all the hospitals to which you have decided to apply (probably ten or more), ranking them in the order of preference. Your school's dean will send this list to a central computer. As the year goes on, and the hospitals make decisions about applicants, they will send their lists of acceptances to the same computer. The computer then matches the applications to the acceptances, giving the students' choices priority. In other words, you will be matched to the hospital highest on your list which chooses you.

You may take your internship in a hospital that has a close affiliation with a medical school, or one whose affiliation is more limited, or one that has only a graduate affiliation—that is, a hospital which takes interns and residents, but does not use its cases for the training of undergraduate medical students. In addition, there are hospitals which have no affiliation at all, but which employ a Director of Medical Education to supervise a program for interns and residents. While these are sometimes good training institutions, it is generally true that the more closely a hospital is affiliated with a medical school, the better its training will be.

There are three kinds of internship: straight, rotating, or rotating-with-emphasis. In a straight internship, you work in one specialty all year. This can be internal medicine (the disorders of the internal organs), surgery, pediatrics, pathology (the study of diseased tissues), obstetrics-gynecology, or family practice (like general practice, but with graduate training including special psychosocial skills). A rotating internship is broken up into six two-month segments, one for each specialty. A rotating-with-emphasis internship falls between the two, with four or more months spent in one specialty. Because of the

A pediatric intern at work. The accomplishments of women in medicine are now being recognized at all levels: this woman was honored by a pediatric society as being the best intern for 1977.

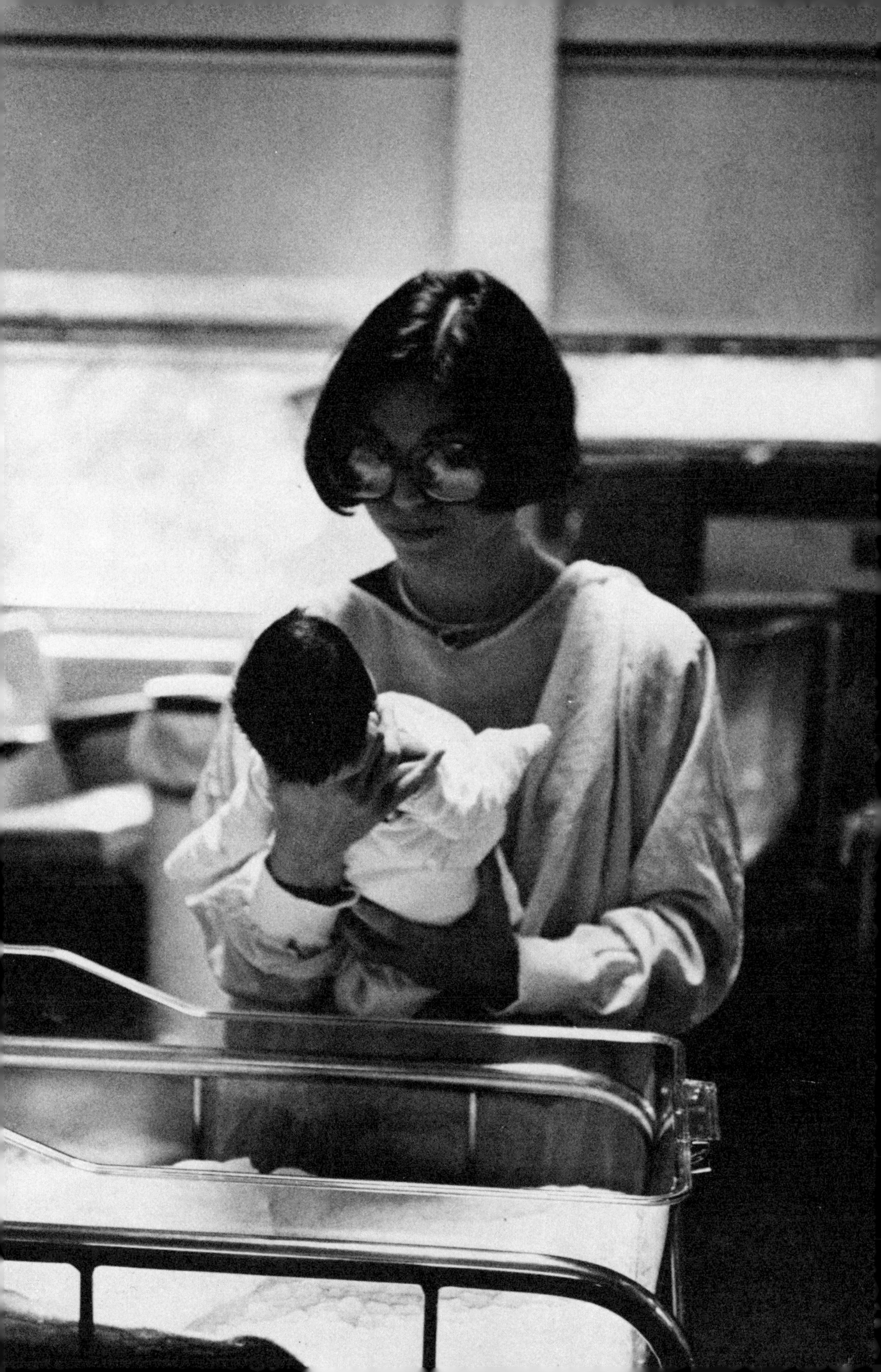

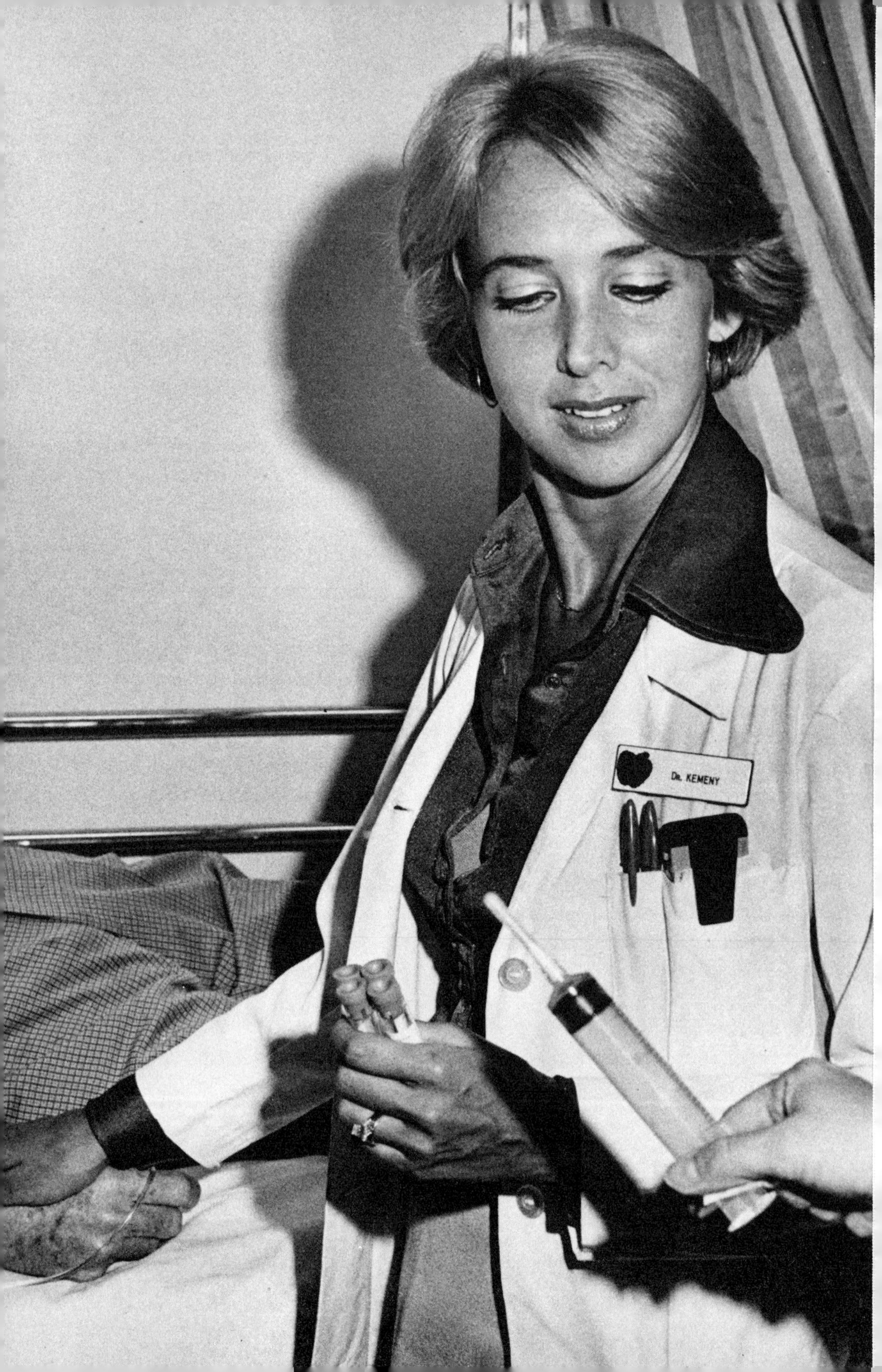
Dr. KEMENY

enormous amounts of knowledge being added to medical science each year, the increasing tendency is for doctors to begin specializing earlier in their careers, and as a result the rotating internship is slowly being phased out. The most prestigious teaching hospitals have abolished it completely, and as of 1972–1973 only 15 percent of all internships in this country were so designated. There are certain circumstances under which a rotating internship might be advisable—if you have not made up your mind about your specialty, for example, or if you know that your future training is going to be so very specialized that your internship will be your last chance to be exposed to a broad spectrum of cases. Still, it is generally agreed that the straight internship is both the preferred and the best kind of first-year graduate work.

The third phase of medical training is the residency. Despite its name, the NIRMP is not generally used for placement in residencies. This is traditionally done on a one-to-one basis between the applicant and the institution. There is an increasing tendency for hospitals to coordinate their internship and residency programs, so that more and more physicians now go from one program to the other without changing location. This is not universal, however, nor does it mean that acceptance to a residency is automatic in such a situation. Most residencies are two or three years in length, although they may be somewhat longer for the surgical specialists.

Residents form the house staff of the hospitals at which they work. All those in a given specialty are supervised by a chief resident, who is chosen from among the last-year residents by

Doctors sometimes must provide care for people who are frightened, anxious, or on the verge of death. They have to be able to handle the pressure, be able to give the desperately needed support to others. This doctor works in cancer chemotherapy. Most of her patients are terminal cases.

the faculty member in charge of that specialty—the "service chief." In hospitals with what is called a "pyramidal structure," where some residents are dropped each year, the selection is made on the basis of merit and is considered a signal honor—medical schools recruit their junior faculty from among such people. In other hospitals the post may be given to anyone willing and able to run just about everything on the floor.

Whereas there are only six possible areas of specialization for an intern, there are about twenty-six for a resident. Some of these, like pediatric, allergy, and orthopedic surgery, are subdivisions of the earlier specialties. Many more, such as radiology, neurology, and otolaryngology (ear, nose, and throat) are not. (Most people going into these take their internships in internal medicine.) With each year of your residency, you will do increasingly specialized work. Upon completion of your residency, you will be "board-eligible," that is, eligible to take the examination for certification in your specialty. These tests are administered by the American Specialty Boards. Passing this examination does not confer any sort of license, and is not required; it simply certifies that you know a certain (vast) amount about your specialty. Not all physicians choose to take these tests, although, like all other forms of academic credentials, they are becoming more important. If you are planning to go into academic medicine or research, you will certainly need board-certification, and the same probably holds true for the private physician who seeks admitting privileges at a good hospital. If you so choose, you can go still further and become board-certified in a *sub*-specialty (if one exists in your field). Examples of these are pulmonary and cardiovascular

After completing medical school, this third year resident took time off to raise a family. Thirteen years later, she returned to complete her specialized work in radiology.

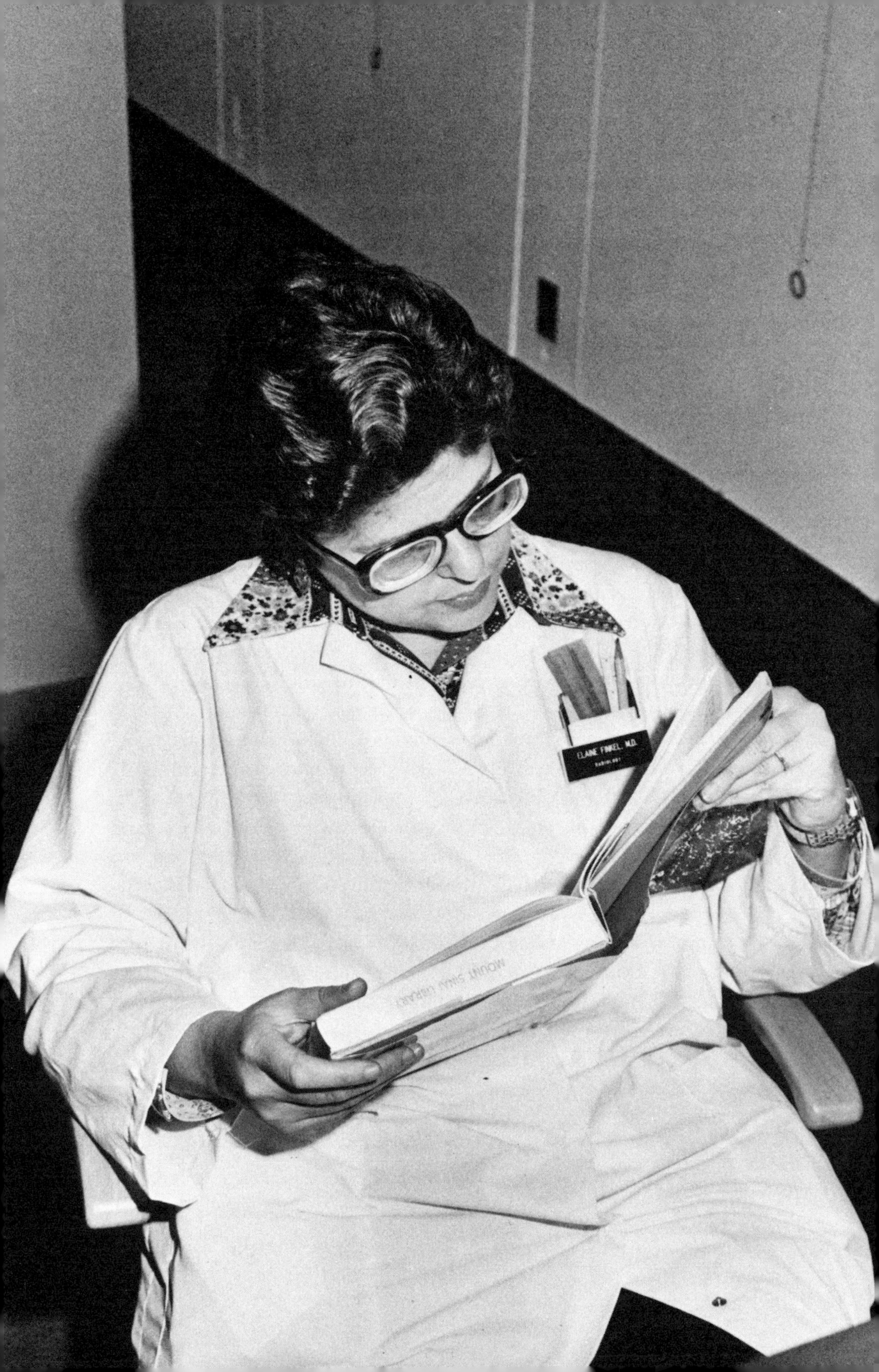
ELAINE FINKEL, M.D.
MOUNT SINAI LIBRARY

disease, endocrinology, and gastroenterology, all of which are subdivisions of internal medicine. To be eligible for this exam, you must have completed a fellowship (usually two years) in that sub-specialty after your residency is over.

Such are the broad outlines of the years of preparation for a medical career. But what does it feel like? Sonya, who had just finished her first year of medical school and had enjoyed it, nevertheless stated that it had reminded her more of junior high school than anything else. "I used my mind far more in college," she explained. "Both high school and college taught me to think and to extrapolate. The first year of medical school is something of a throwback." While the first two years do contain the bulk of the classroom work you will encounter in medical school—textbooks, lectures, and memorization—most schools have begun combining these elements with clinical instruction on the hospital floors so that students may have an immediate opportunity to apply what they learn in the classroom. However, full-time clinical learning does not begin until the third year.

The third year of medical school is divided into periods called "rotations" or "clerkships," each devoted to a different basic specialty: internal medicine (often simply called "medicine," a term confusing to many laymen), surgery, pediatrics, and obstetrics-gynecology. In tandem with a small group of classmates, you will make the rounds of the wards, always under the supervision of faculty members and house staff. The doctors in charge will discuss each case with you and will request your professional opinion. You will receive a grade in each of these clerkships, issued for the benefit of the hospitals to which you will be applying for internships in your senior year.

For Linda, a Midwesterner studying medicine in New York, the on-the-spot give-and-take of third-year work required not only a new way of thinking, but a new way of acting as well. "In the third year clerkships, everything is run in small groups where you're graded on aggressiveness. You have to change your personality. I encountered my first sexism that year—before, it was just dumb jokes."

And what about sexism in medical school? It would be unrealistic to say that it does not exist, but it is not easy to generalize about it. Some students say they never experienced it at all; others recall it with bitterness. Where you are is one factor. There are schools (New York University Medical School is one) which are known to be liberal in their attitudes toward female applicants and students (there can, of course, be a few exceptions on the faculties in these places). Then there are schools which have a reputation for being difficult for women—Cornell and Harvard are examples. Your personal experience will also depend on the nature of your fellow students, and on which professors you draw. The number of women in your class is something else that can make a difference, at least as far as moral support is concerned.

You might want to look up a book entitled *Why Would a Girl Go into Medicine?* by Margaret A. Campbell, M.D. (Feminist Press, Old Westbury, 1973). Dr. Campbell (a pseudonym) sent out questionnaires to women at 41 medical schools, asking for their experiences. Since the research was addressed entirely to the matter of sex discrimination, you might get the feeling while reading the book that that is the *only* experience that women have in medical school. Obviously that is not the case. However, the fact that the problem clearly does exist is enough to warrant a brief examination of the three main sources of sex discrimination: the faculty, the students, and the physical set-up of the medical school.

Linda's experience with her faculty surgery chief was typical of one extreme. On rounds he had been asking her many more questions than he asked anyone else, and she finally asked him why. "Well, somebody's got to pick on the cute little blonde," he replied in a reasonable tone. At the other end of the spectrum, a number of Campbell's respondents complained, not of being harassed, but of being completely ignored. The word "Gentlemen," used to address a class which includes women, eventually proves intolerable. Then there is the very common complaint of *Playboy*-type photos being included in the carousel of slides that are used in pathology lectures. One professor accused of this practice by a female student reportedly replied, "Men have to look down on women, and that's why I show those slides." However, there may well be another factor contributing to this practice, one that has been suggested by teachers and students alike. It can take a certain amount of emotional stamina to watch an hour's worth of photographs of diseased tissue without losing one's professional cool, at least at the beginning of training. When, at the end of a lecture, a voluptuous female nude flashes unexpectedly across the screen, the male students at least are finally able to express a shared emotional reaction. That kind of release can be therapeutic—for the men, if not for their female classmates.

As for the male students, some of them may have trouble accepting the idea of a woman becoming a doctor—especially right in their very midst. "Every time women were mentioned in a class discussion, all heads would swing around toward me, and *I hated that,*" Carol remembers. "There I was, the sole representative of womankind, that exotic species." This situation has become less acute, however, as female medical students become less exotic every year.

The problems arising from physical arrangements in medical school buildings stem from the fact that such buildings traditionally have had their dressing rooms, sleeping quarters, bathrooms, etc., labeled not "Men" and "Women," but "Doctors" or "Medical Students" and "Nurses." As a result, every medical student who is *not* a man has at least one locker-room story. For example, Carol reports as follows:

> "I'd gone to change into my whites early, before anyone else had arrived for rounds. I went into the room marked 'Medical Students' and left my stuff in a locker. When I came back after work, I found the room full of men in various stages of undress. One guy was really furious. He yelled at me, 'Can't you read?

The sign on the door says "Men"!' " Carol took him outside and showed him what the sign on the door really said.

"Oh," he said.

"For him," Carol concluded, "it *did* say 'Men.' "

The last year of medical school was described by one graduate as something of a cross between the third year and the internship. During the fourth year you might take a junior internship in your chosen specialty, or enter an elective clinical or research program, and then, almost immediately after graduation, you will begin duty as an intern.

Being an intern is a uniquely concentrated medical experience. One physician compared it to the puberty rites primitive tribes require of their young braves to prove their valor. It is probably unlike anything you will ever do again. Lisa described her year as follows:

"You come in at eight in the morning and leave at six the next night. The next day, you're on duty from eight to six. Then, the day after that, you do thirty-six hours again. You see, interns are the only people on active duty at night. The residents sleep in the hospital too, but they're not on call for that kind of routine thing—they're more like supervisors. You handle all the night admissions and decide what has to be done. You do all the physical procedures—intravenous, electrocardiograms, taking off casts, blood spinning. In a way, it's a boring year, with a lot of technical, repetitive work. You don't have to be a genius, you just have to be compulsive. Until an emergency comes up—then you have to remember everything you know about that particular problem."

Lisa summed up her internship as "the worst year of my life—and the best."

"I've developed as a mature human being. It's changed my whole value system. I'm not the same person anymore. I've seen so many sad things—young people dying . . . You never get over something like that. It makes you value every minute you're alive and feeling pretty good. I always used to take life for granted.

"And it's true that people's lives really do depend on you. I've saved lives this year. There's no other experience like that in the world."

Over the past few years attempts have been made to phase out the internship year, on the grounds that the senior year of medical school supplies enough of that sort of experience, and that an internship is simply one more year of the same. In fact, in 1973 over a thousand medical school graduates were admitted directly into residencies, most of these being in surgery (the longest residency) and psychiatry (for which a straight internship no longer exists). Virtually no experienced physicians consider this a good idea. "You need that extra year to acclimatize yourself to responsibility," was the way one summed it up. "It's not something you can get any other way." Lisa's words would seem to demonstrate how, in one sense, this is profoundly true. In agreement with this is Betty, speaking from the vantage point of her last year of residency:

"I remember how it suddenly all came together for the first time—medicine is really exciting that way. I'd never had a sense of my own competence before. Suddenly I was thinking about the *why* of what I was doing, not just wondering what decision my service chief would want me to make. That was the real turning point in my training. Before that time, I never thought I'd have enough faith in myself to take the responsibility for people's lives. Now I know I can, and I do."

Residency is still an important part of training; in the second and third years especially, you will be working in your specialty, which increases intellectual responsibility. Judy, who was a resident in neurology, remembered that "a lot of internists don't know that much neurology, and they don't always recognize the syndromes. You've got to keep your eyes open and be ready to point things out. They argue a little bit harder about it when you're a girl; you just have to argue back—

loudly. The main thing is to keep your feet on the ground and not get hysterical—then they'll see you can handle it."

Residents are also administrators, especially in hospitals with no pyramidal structure. They essentially run the work of the floor, making up schedules for patient care, deciding when patients are to be discharged, and apportioning the work. There was a time when they actually "resided" in the hospitals full-time, eating and sleeping there, and being on call at nights, weekends, even on vacations—all for practically no money. Those days are over. Now, although they still sleep in the hospital a certain number of nights a week, they have time off and they do get a salary—in 1976, it averaged just under $14,000 a year in affiliated hospitals, and just over that sum in non-affiliated ones. (Interns get paid for their year too, about a thousand dollars less in each case.) Non-affiliated hospitals are able to pay slightly higher wages because they don't have to contribute to the salaries of a medical school faculty.

Important also is the fact that residents teach. Not only do they supervise the work of the interns under them, making the more sophisticated decisions for them when that is necessary, they work with junior and senior medical school students as well. For some residents, this is the most rewarding part. "The house staff gets jaded with the years," one resident commented, "but to the medical students it's all new. They're fresher and more idealistic. It's more fun to work with them." Every year a few women in each hospital will feel this way, and decide to make the teaching of medicine all or a part of their life's work. In the next chapter we will see what it is like for them.

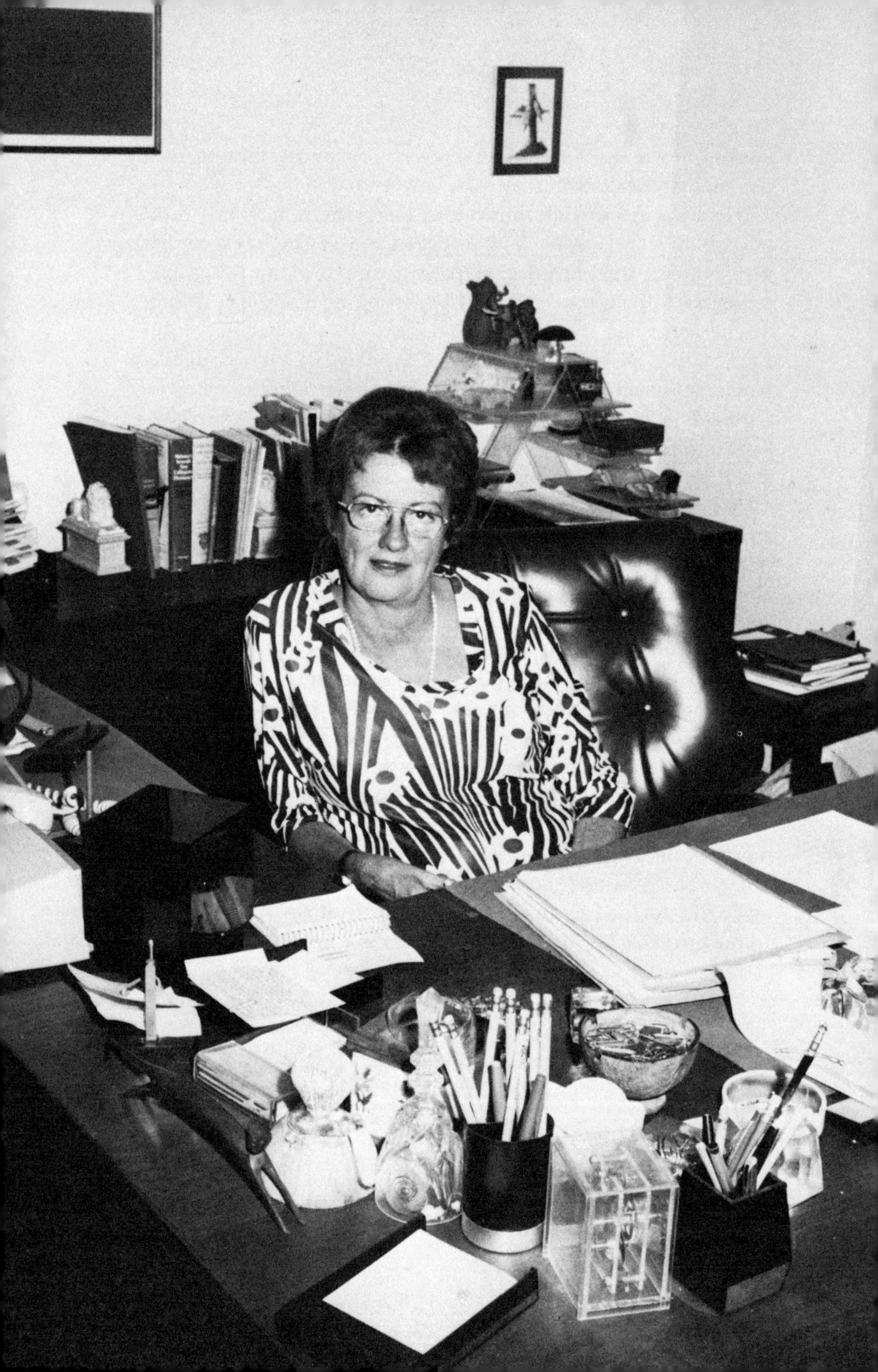

4

Academic Medicine

If you ask any woman who teaches medicine what she likes best about it, she will probably tell you, "Learning so much from the students."

"I find it very demanding and very refreshing," said one psychiatrist in her sixties, whose enthusiasm was typical. "I feel challenged. I learn from it. There's no end to what you have to learn."

In fact, you may have to run to keep up. "Today's medical students have no reticence about asking questions or making challenges," one pathologist said. "They feel free. This forces a teacher to examine her own feelings, her own point of view. They ask me many questions and demand the latest answers. Sometimes they've read something I haven't. There's a lot of give and take."

There are two kinds of instructors at medical schools—academic and clinical. Academic professors work mostly in classrooms, teaching pathology and the medical specialties. Clinical professors are the ones who take students, interns, and residents on rounds through the hospital, demonstrating how physicians recognize and diagnose a disease, and handle patients. A number of women in clinical teaching emphasized the need to search constantly for more effective ways to present the actual practice of medicine to their students. One said, "I see the role as an introduction to relating to patients, an introduction to what goes on outside of school. A doctor has very important decisions to make once she gets out there in the world. To prepare her for that, you've got to give her not just facts, but approaches."

There are not many women in academic medicine in the United States—the estimated number as of September 1972 was 4,200, a small percentage of all the people on medical faculties at that time, although it was considerably larger than what you would have found in most European countries. Also, while the number of women teaching medicine is increasing all the time, it is still quite difficult for a woman to rise past a certain point in the academic ranks. Indeed, the female service head, in charge of a whole department, is extremely rare.

In view of all this, it is interesting to consider the results of a study of "Women Physicians on US Medical School Faculties," published by H. P. Jolly in the *Journal of Medical Education* in August of 1975. Jolly found that in almost every year from 1940 to 1970, a larger percentage of the women who graduated from medical school went into teaching than was the case among their male colleagues. (Since prior to 1965 women accounted for something under ten percent of all medical graduates, they still remained a definite minority among medical professors, despite their apparent greater proclivity for the work.) Women also showed a slightly greater tendency to enter the academic ranks of medical faculties than did men, although this was not the case in the somewhat less prestigious

This psychiatrist both maintains a private practice and teaches in a large city hospital where her students get a chance to benefit from her years of experience.

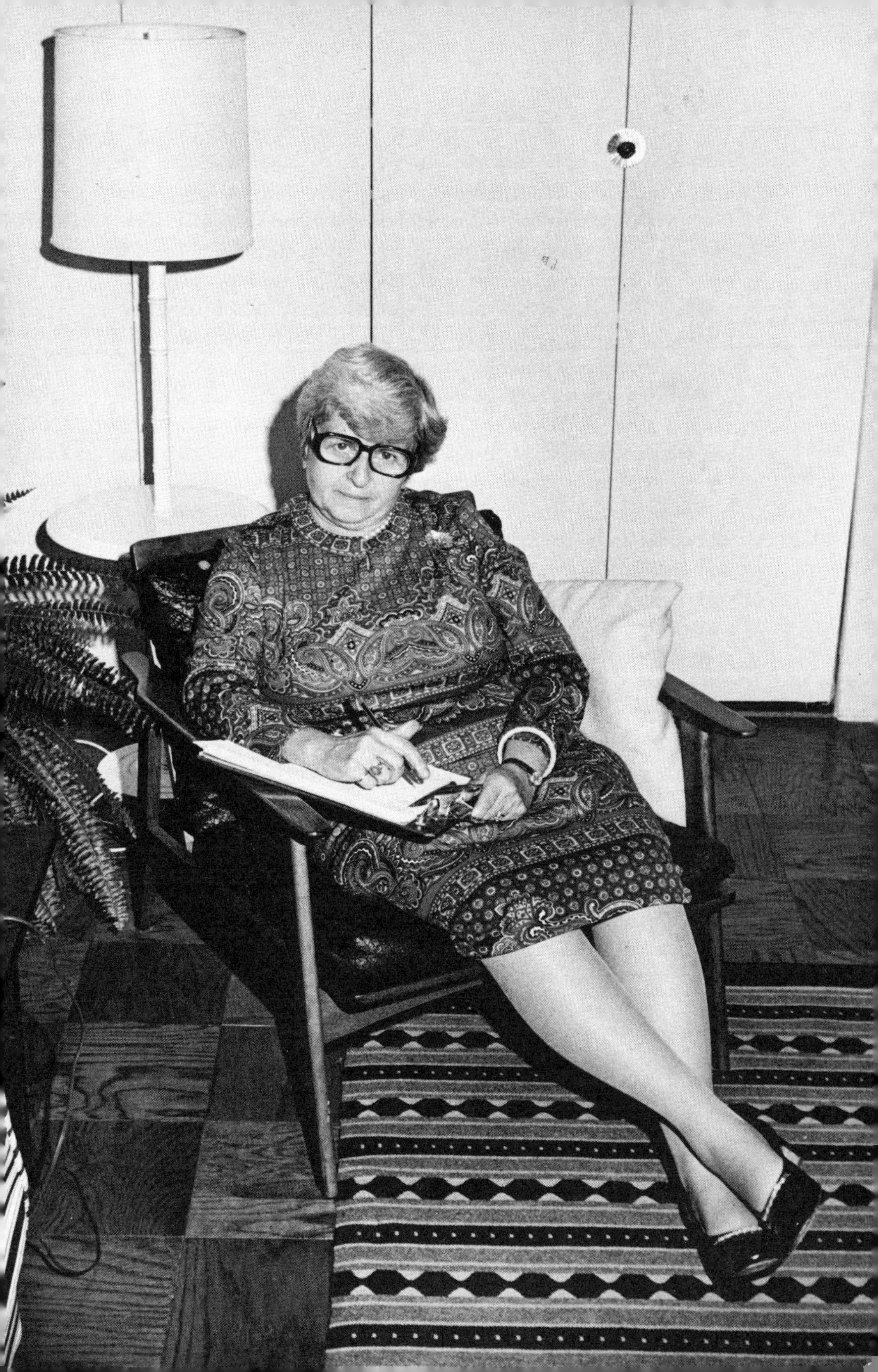

clinical sphere. This may be due to the fact that while an academic professor will almost certainly have a full-time institutional commitment, a clinical professor will be also—or primarily—a private practitioner, devoting only some of her time to going on rounds. Since women tend to go into private practice less frequently than men, primarily because the irregularity of the hours can conflict with the demands of a home and family, they consequently prefer full-time institutional work.

And of course there is the question of money. A working woman married to a man who also works does not have to worry about her salary to quite the same extent as a man who has to support his whole family by himself. Academic professors are well paid—they get about twice as much money as professors in colleges and universities—but they still do not make as much as clinical professors. This is due to the fact that, even though clinical professors are paid less by the medical school, they can more than make up the difference from their own private practices. Most people on medical faculties fall into this category—they are part-time instructors who take a certain percentage of their working hours—usually less than half—away from their practices to teach on hospital floors. The most common minimum commitment for such people involves going on rounds for two or three months every year, in return for which they are allowed to admit their patients to the hospital ("admitting privileges") when necessary. When that happens, those patients also become teaching cases, about whom their doctor will lecture the students and house staff. In a big city, with a large medical center, any board-certified specialist in private practice will probably have a faculty appointment of at least this kind.

There are two other categories of teaching physicians in addition to the part-time contingent: full-time (or geographical full-time) and full-full-time (also called strict full-time). A faculty member who does geographical full-time work will continue to see a number of private patients, but she will see them only on the hospital premises (hence the idea of geography).

A strict full-time professor will be involved in nothing except teaching and research. This last group are the most powerful and prestigious people in the medical school. It is from their ranks that the service chiefs are drawn. They may occasionally see a private patient or two, but when they do, they are required to turn over their earnings to the hospital, which has already taken the responsibility for their full income. Otherwise they have no direct patient responsibility, although, like geographical full-time people, they have the indirect responsibility of being attending house physicians ("attendings" for short). This means that they supervise the work of the house staff and are available for consultation should a patient's private physician wish to call on them.

There are two exceptions to this, however: A staff attending can have the opportunity to treat patients individually if she works in a hospital clinic, or if there is a municipal hospital affiliated with her school. A clinic is an outpatient (or "ambulatory care") unit in a hospital, where patients go for the treatment of problems not serious enough to warrant hospitalization. Such a clinic may be either general or specialized. Its patients may have been referred by someone in the hospital itself, or they may have come for a second opinion about something, or they may have merely walked in off the street. The house staff and attendings who work there meet and treat these patients in the same way a doctor in a private office would. Many find this situation very attractive. One young woman in immunology research, for example, works in three clinics a week, partly because it is the only chance she gets to see patients directly. She does not plan to go into private practice because she prefers the academic sphere, but she intends to do clinic work on the side whenever possible. "I like to see patients very much," she said. "I'm not working in a lab because I don't!"

As for municipal, or publicly supported hospitals, the patients in them have not been admitted by a private physician usually because they could not afford to go to one. They have come via the emergency room, or have been brought in by an

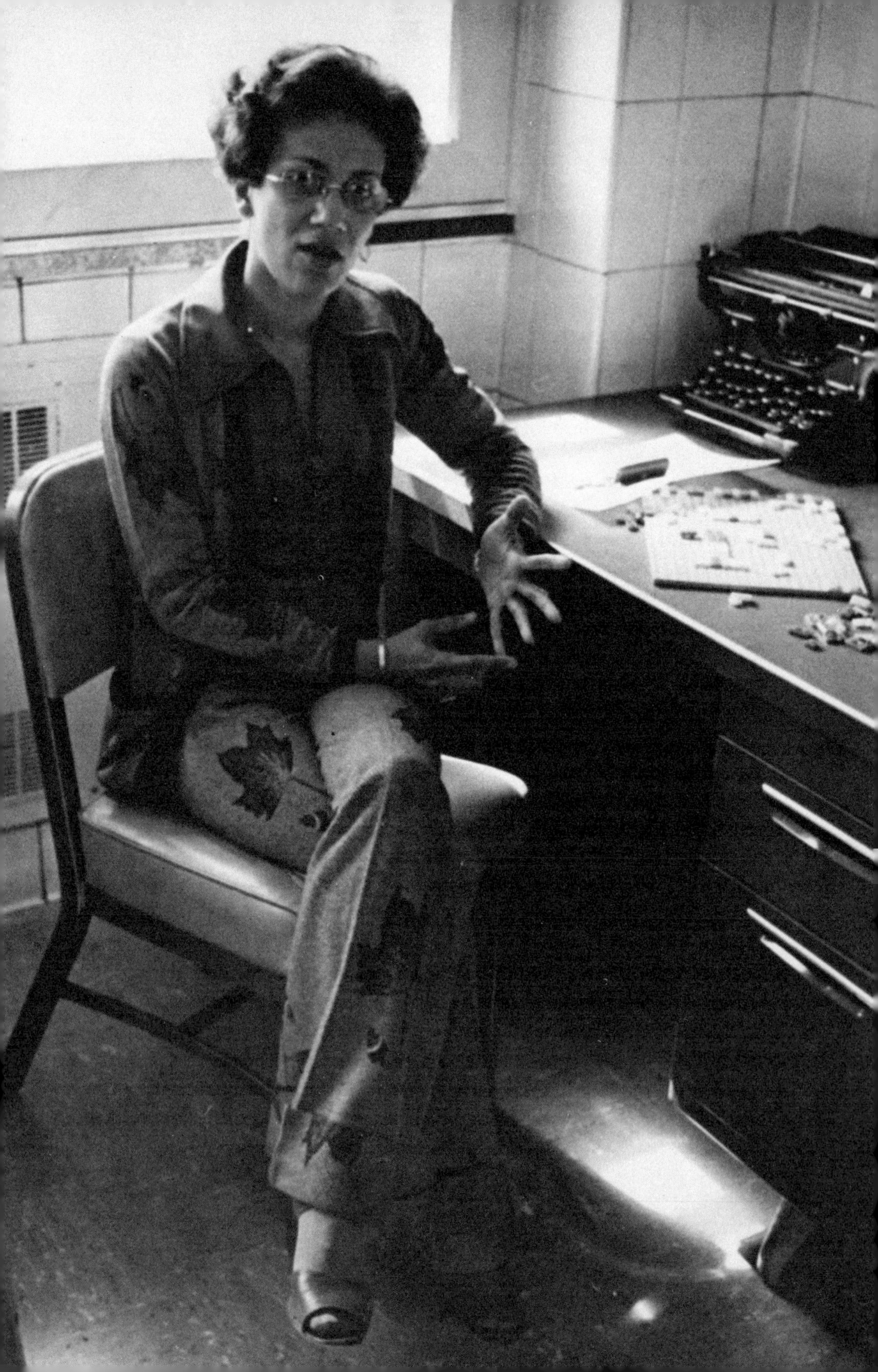

ambulance. Therefore, the only doctors treating them will be those on the house staff, or attendings from the affiliated school. Most medical schools in big cities number at least one municipal hospital among their affiliated houses, used especially for this purpose. The patients are very poor and the settings are not elegant—there are no private or semi-private rooms, only long wards full of beds. Still, one doctor reported she preferred the hours put in at her municipal hospital to the ones she spent in the much more luxurious private institution also connected with her school. "It's because I have the actual jurisdiction there," she explained. "With private admissions, I can only advise the house staff. But when I work with the service admissions here, I actually make the decisions about patient care. I spend most of my time in the lab and that's something I don't often get the chance to do."

But, as keen as the conflict between the desire to treat patients and to do research can be, physicians in the academic sphere do not generally regret whatever they might be missing of patient responsibility. They are in the most intellectually prestigious and demanding part of the whole medical profession, and they love it. They love the wealth of challenging, complex problems they get to deal with by being based in a hospital, and they love the intellectual stimulation of being in an environment whose whole purpose is to learn and to discover.

Work in medicine can be extremely varied. This doctor, as an administrator, is Deputy Chief of Child Psychiatry at a public hospital, and Director of the Child and Adolescent Psychiatric Day Hospital. She is also a teacher, supervising interns and medical school students, and a child psychiatrist, providing care for the children at her hospital.

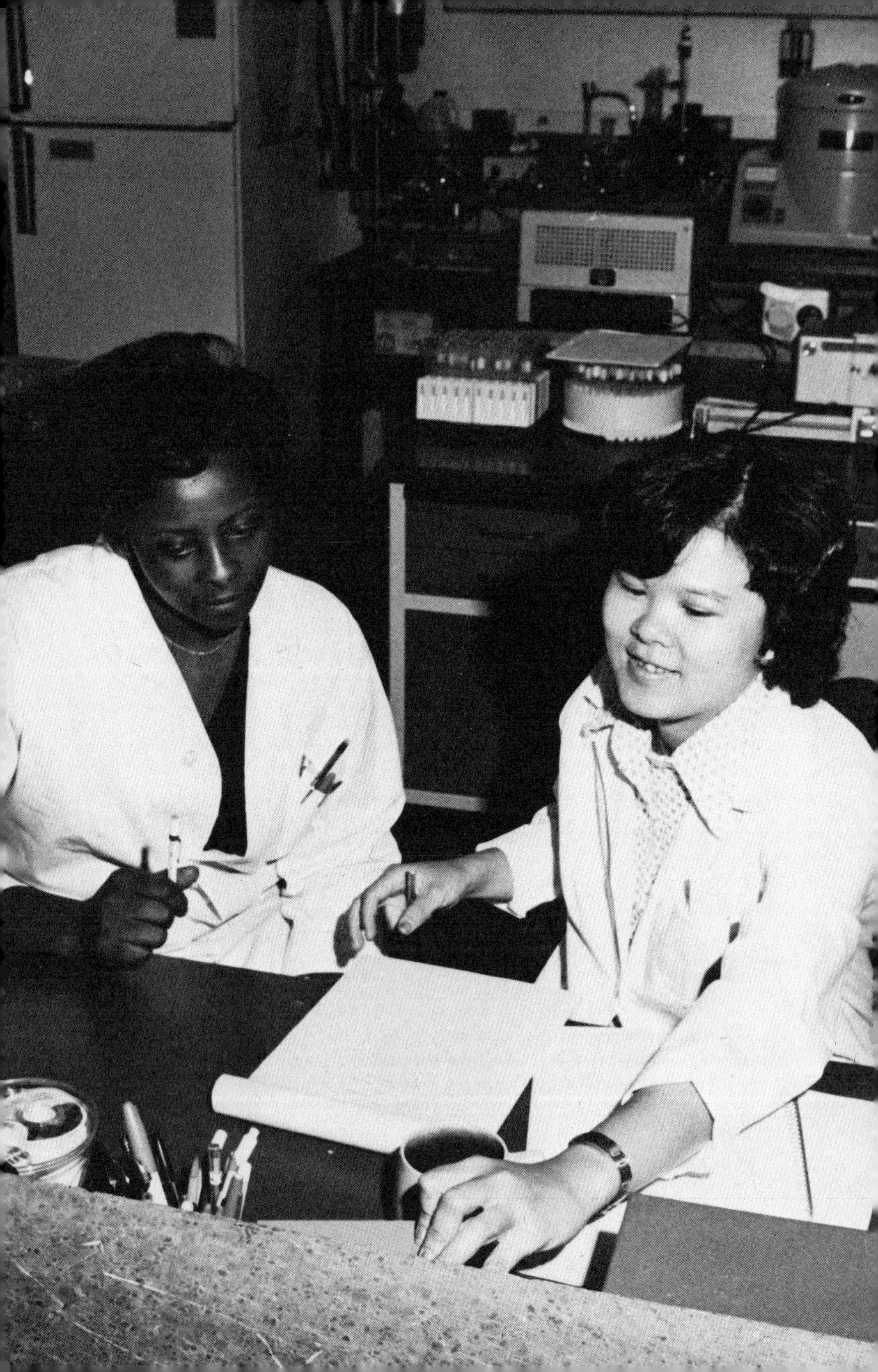

5

Research

The saying "publish or perish," which rules the academic world at large, holds true in medicine as well. Because of this, the doctor who decides to make academic medicine most or all of her professional life is going to be doing research work as well. She must do so in order to maintain her professional reputation (and, possibly, her job), and she will have to publish her findings with some regularity in order to continue the flow of grant money which makes the work possible. Do not, however, get the idea that most doctors engaged in research regard it simply as necessary drudgery. On the contrary, most of them love it. They love the intellectual stimulation it provides, the way it satisfies their curiosity while at the same time encouraging them to pursue further questions, and they especially enjoy the thrill of discovering something no one ever knew before. Those who have been involved in research, and then had to give it up because of the pressure of other commitments, generally look back on it fondly—even wistfully. One woman who pursued research did so because she remembered how frustrated her father had been at the way his private practice eventually took over his whole professional life, leaving him no time for the laboratory.

There are two opinions on this issue, however, and if patient contact and pure clinical work are what you enjoy most, then it will be laboratory work that will frustrate you most. One woman who now works in a Veterans' Administration hospital, for example, left Rockefeller University after three years' work with animals in the immunology lab. She had enjoyed it, but she missed talking to patients, and she wanted to feel that she was doing something which related more immediately to people. In general, however, it is probably safe to assume that if you feel drawn to academic medicine, the same things you find attractive there will also make research satisfying to you. One woman, putting it as simply as possible, said, "It's fun, because you're finding out new things."

You find out new things by asking questions—but you have to know *how* to ask. "You have to have a formulated curiosity," one woman said. "You have to have *questions,* all the time; you've got to have the kind of mind that looks at the world and never stops wondering why things happen. And you have to have the intellectual apparatus, the learning in your field, that will enable you to pursue your questions to the end. Or to the answer at least. There's never really any end."

Research is commonly said to fall into two categories, clinical and laboratory, although there is some overlap. In its most elementary form, clinical research can simply mean writing up a report of a new case, for example, one containing a combination of symptoms never before observed together. Most clinical research concerns the effects of new drugs on diseases which have so far resisted treatment, such as cancer and kidney

This doctor has enormous enthusiasm for her work. Her research in cellular immunology may contribute to a better understanding of leukemia.

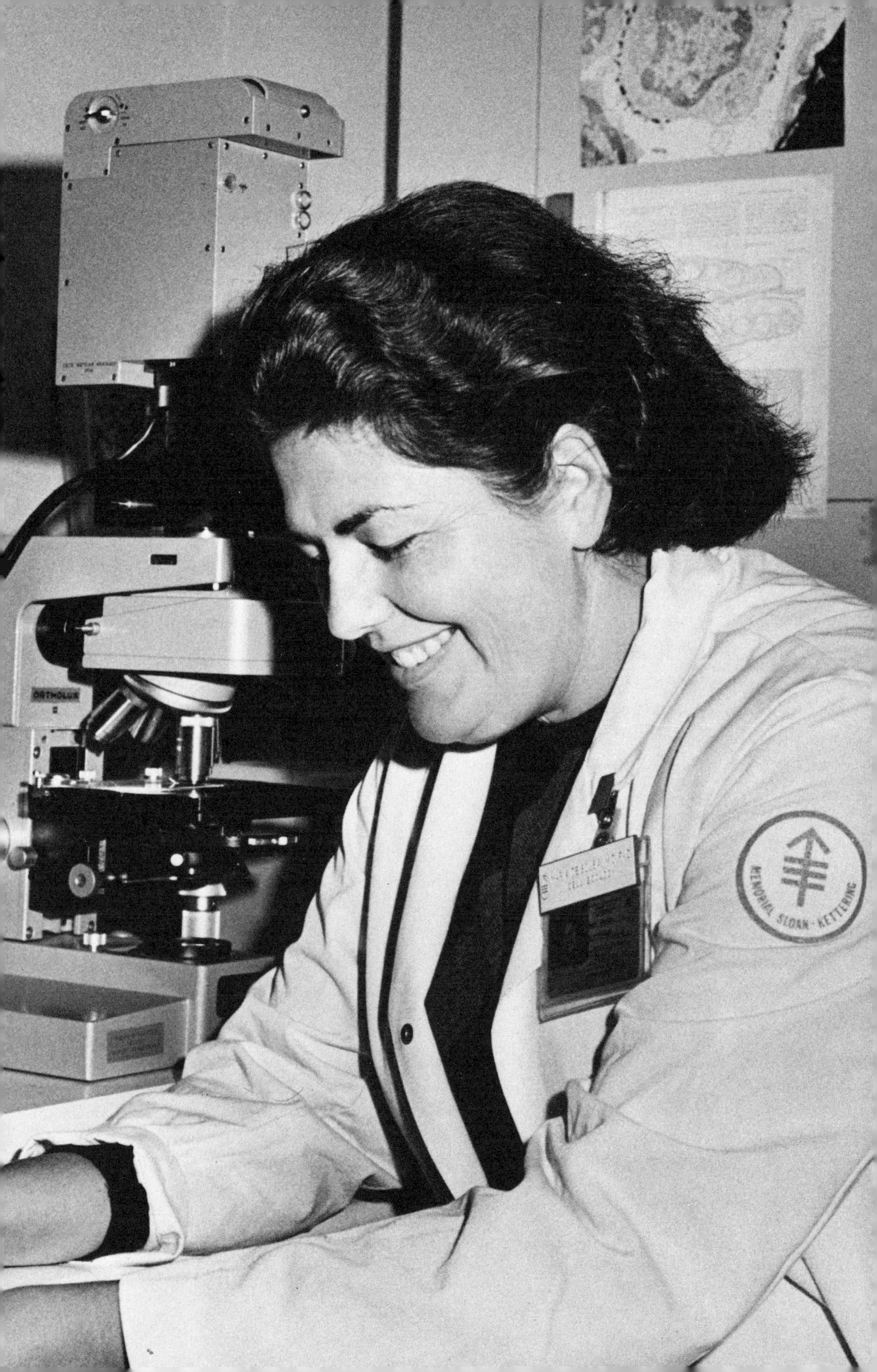
ORTHOLUX
MEMORIAL SLOAN-KETTERING

disease. "Double-blind" studies are often used, meaning that neither the patients nor the doctors know which patients are getting the drug under study, and which are getting the placebo which is the control in the experiment. Thus the results cannot be distorted by anyone's expectations.

Lab research involves a great deal of work with animals. One large teaching hospital has an entire floor inhabited by cats, dogs, sheep, goats, chickens, rabbits, and several armies of white mice. A whole branch of veterinary medicine, called lab animal work, is devoted to raising these animals and seeing to it that the federal laws requiring their humane treatment are adhered to. Medical research as we know it would have been impossible without these animals. They are not only used for determining the effects and side effects of drugs, however. One woman who had addressed most of her professional life to the study of children's growth had a large selection of white rats in her laboratory which she used in experiments concerning the effects of hormones on development. Also, not all research uses animals—sometimes the object of study can be a single cell. One doctor working in cellular immunology, a relatively new field, was studying the effects of depleting the populations of lymphocytes, whose job it is to protect the body against disease. Another studied the effects of hormones on individual cells. Still another was working exclusively with chemical models, analyzing the nutritive elements of protein. Laboratory or "bench" work at this end of the research spectrum, as far away from immediate practical applicability to patients as one can get, is called the most "basic" kind of research.

Lab research often centers on work with animals. Here, mice are being used for immunogenetic investigations. On the basis of her reputation, this researcher was honored with an invitation to attend a special program at the Sorbonne, where she received the equivalent of the American Ph.D.

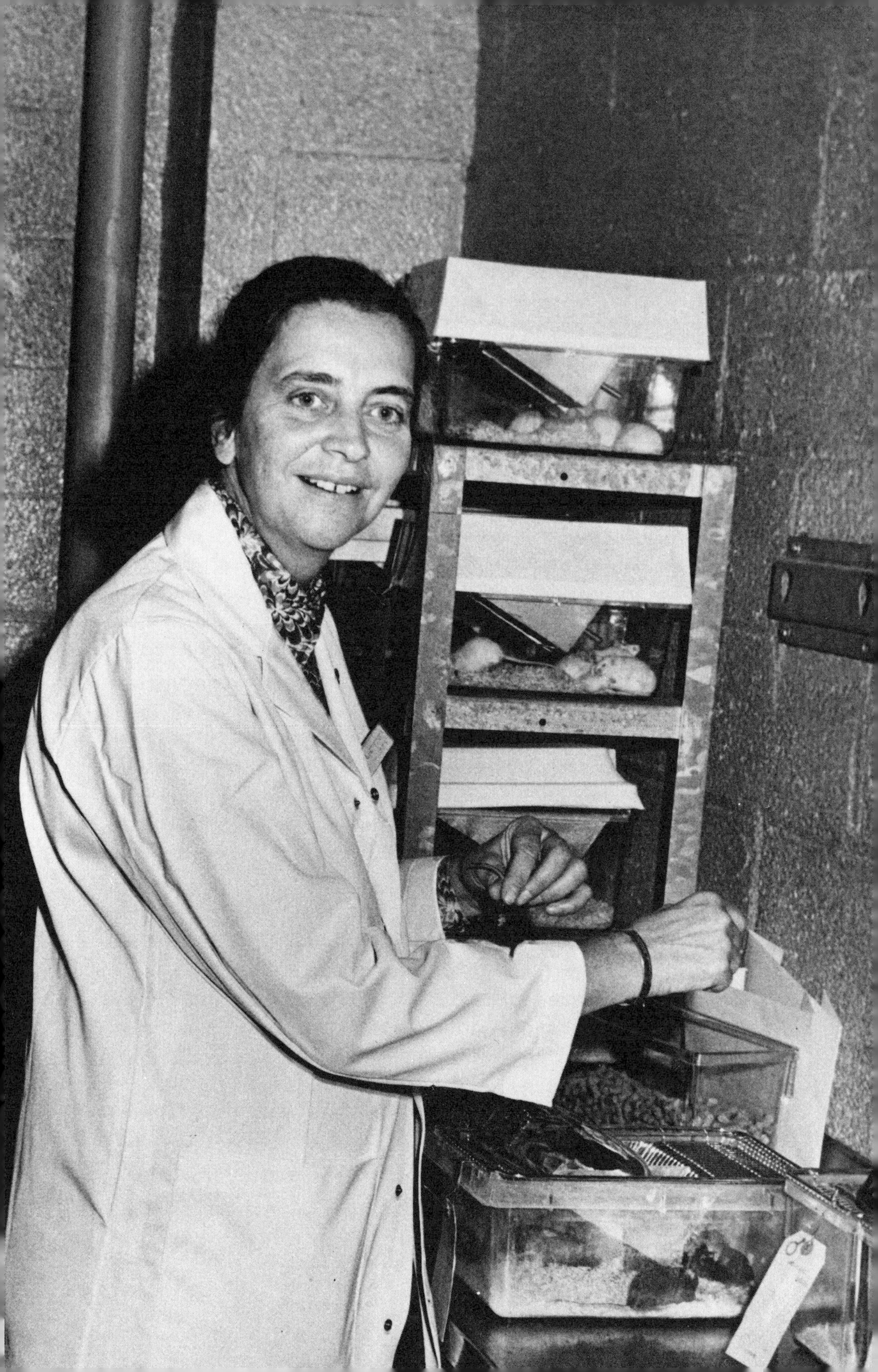

Research is almost never a full-time occupation for a physician. It is usually mixed in varying proportions with her academic and clinical commitments. It can be carried out in the wards and laboratories of the hospitals where she works, but the money the researcher needs—for equipment, assistants' salaries, and living expenses—will come, not from the institution itself, but from the government via the National Institute of Health (NIH), which administers all federal funds earmarked for medical research—now about $2.2 billion annually.

The mention of such funds brings us to the subject of grant applications. The word most often used to describe these by doctors who have gone through them is "horrible." "You have to fit yourself into their mold," was the way one woman described the process. "You have to tell them exactly what you want to find out from the research. Well, that's not hard. But you have to tell them *exactly how* you're going to do it, and that's something you can't always know at the outset. Exactly how many assistants, for exactly how long, exactly what equipment, and exactly how long each phase will take you. You see these gray hairs? Each one is a page of a grant application!" One woman left research because she felt she could put her time to better use than filling out those pages and pages of forms. Most doctors, however, accept it as a necessary evil, and stick it out. "It's just a part of your work, after all," one said stoically. "If you really can't stand it, you do something else instead."

After it has been submitted, an application has to go through an exhaustive process known as "peer review" to determine whether the project will qualify for funding. The NIH votes favorably on about 11,000 research projects a year, at a cost of $676 million. The money allocated is actually given, not to the individual, but to the institution with which she is affiliated, which then in turn pays for and monitors her work.

The NIH, however, is not simply an agency for the disbursement of government funds—it is itself a huge research institute, one of the most prestigious in the world. Situated on

306 acres in Bethesda, Md., about 10 miles from Washington, D.C., it employs 13,000 workers, of whom approximately 1,000 are doctors, dentists, and veterinarians. It is actually made up of twelve separate institutes, each set up for the study of a different field: cancer, heart and lung disease, aging, allergy and infectious diseases, arthritis, metabolism and digestive disorders, child health and human development, dental research, general medical science, neurological disorders and stroke, ophthalmology, and environmental health (the last is headquartered in North Carolina). There is also the 1,500,000-volume National Library of Medicine, the largest research library in the world devoted to a single subject.

In addition, there is the 516-bed Clinical Center, a hospital whose purpose is actually to serve as a giant research facility. To be admitted, a patient must be suffering from a disease under study—they are referred by physicians all over the country. There is twice as much laboratory space as there is bed space, all of which is set up adjacent to the patients' rooms. Doctors interested in research can apply for work at the Clinical Center after completing the first year of their residency. While there, they will be able to observe any given disease in a great variety of forms, and will have an almost unlimited supply of expert technicians—microbiologists, biochemists, and the like—to talk to about what they see. After two or three years there, they will be among the most eligible applicants for academic posts in the whole country.

There is another kind of medical research that also should be mentioned: the development and testing of drugs for pharmaceutical companies. The process by which a prescription drug is allowed to go on the market in this country—thanks to the rigor of the Food and Drug Administration—requires an application about thirty volumes long, costs about $5 million, and takes about ten years. The claims made in advertising over-the-counter drugs, thanks to the vigilance of the Federal Trade Commission, must be subject to constant testing to re-establish their validity. The work mandated by these regulations

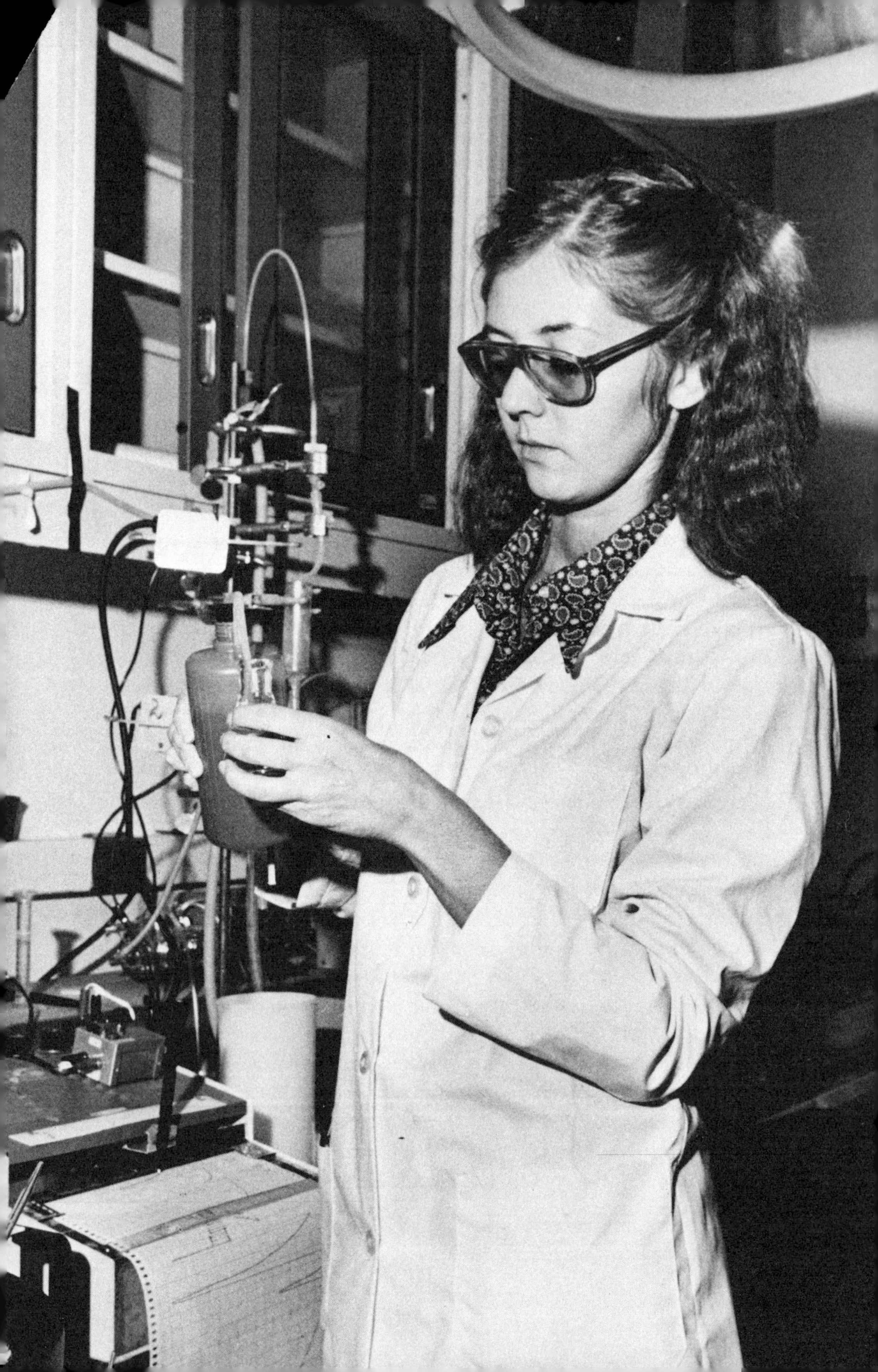

and many more is done by the doctors who work for the various "ethical" or "proprietary" houses currently in the business of making medicine. (Ethical houses make prescription drugs; proprietary ones make products sold over-the-counter.)

Physicians have been known to look down on their colleagues who go to work for drug companies on the grounds that they are selling their talent to people who only want to use it to make money. The work, however, is important. For the woman with a family, there is the advantage of the eight-hour day and the five-day week; for one with more time to spare, there are numerous possibilities for travel. Built into the work is the opportunity to keep abreast of the latest happenings in medical research, something many physicians wish they had time to do more adequately. The one thing you will not have in this field, of course, is contact with patients, but, as with other forms of research, you may well feel that in the end you are having an impact on the health of more people than you could ever physically treat and influence in one lifetime.

The research this doctor is pursuing may ultimately lead to a new pharmacological treatment of heart disease. For a career in research you *must* have patience. Sometimes it takes years to find the answers . . . sometimes a lifetime.

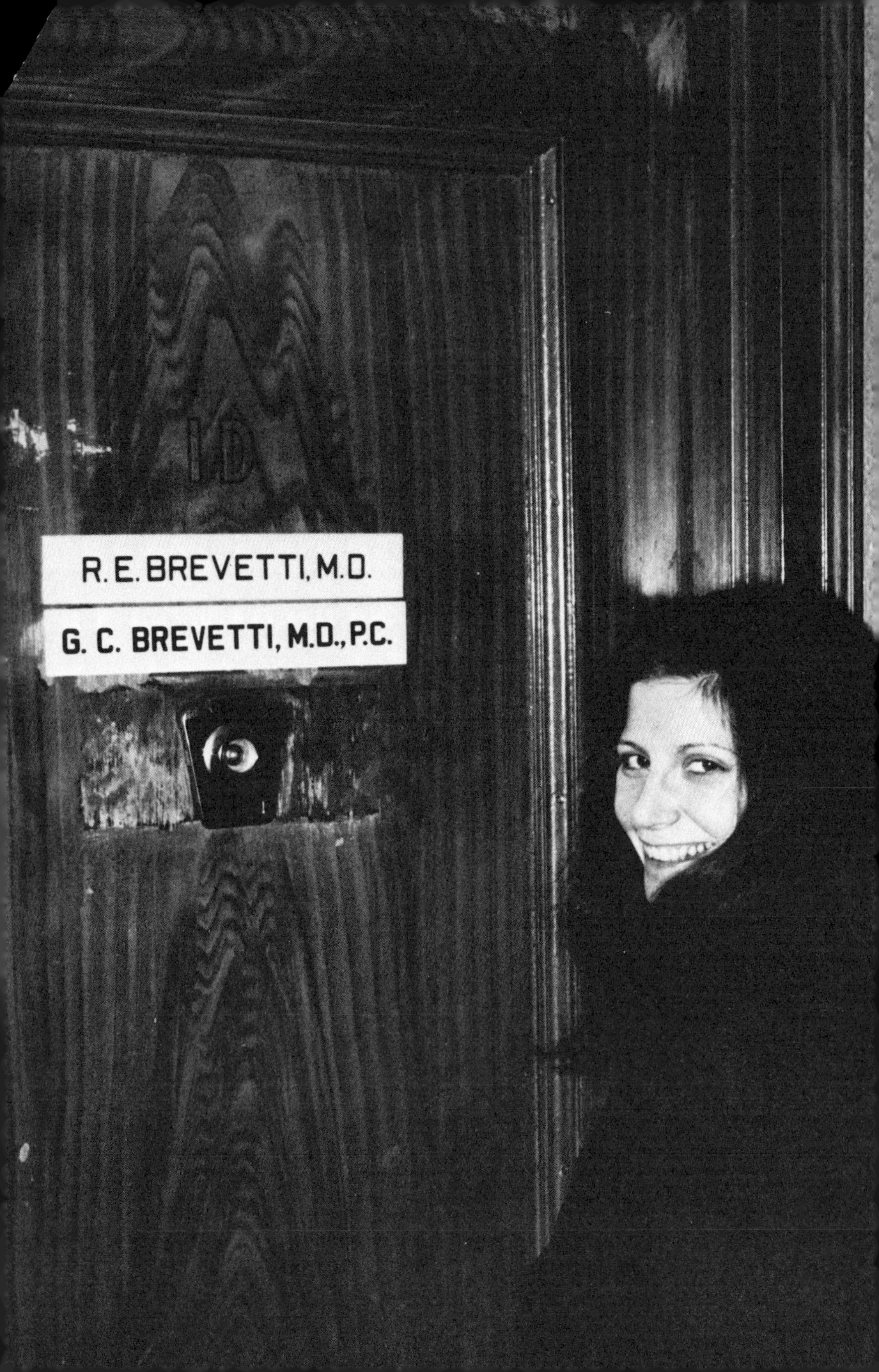
1D
R. E. BREVETTI, M.D.
G. C. BREVETTI, M.D., P.C.

6

Private Practice

Private practice is ideal for the woman who prefers caring for people on a one-to-one relationship over the more academic challenge of research or hospital work. It is for the woman who likes to be her own boss in what is among other things a small-business set-up. It is for the woman who is ready to cope with a work situation where her patients may come in drips and droplets one year, and in an overwhelming flood the next. It is for the woman who is not afraid that the mechanics of a fee-for-service relationship will complicate her role as a ministrant. And it is for someone who is capable of establishing and maintaining good relationships with her colleagues. She will not be working with them in the same way she would in a hospital, but she is going to need their steady professional respect in order to get patient referrals, particularly if she is a specialist just setting up her practice.

Here is how one woman, who worked for thirty years with her husband in a neighborhood general-practice partnership, explained her love for the work: "We had what amounted to a country practice in an urban setting. Over the years we delivered babies to girls we ourselves had delivered years earlier.

As our patients moved away, they'd come back from all over the country to have their check-ups with us! It was *very* satisfying. I still get mail from my old patients every week—good news and bad."

As a general practitioner, this woman cared for whole families. Physicians in specialties also enjoy the benefits of a continuing relationship with their patients—for them, too, it is the chief attraction of the private setting. One dermatologist said, "I like people, which is lucky because otherwise I'd get bored just looking at warts all day. That's why I enjoy private practice. I talk to my patients and get to know them. A clinic is so impersonal."

However, these women never sever their institutional links entirely. Like most private practitioners, they allot a certain part of their time for hospital work and teaching. There are two reasons why this is necessary. One is practical: you will need admitting privileges at a nearby hospital for the times when your patients will need to go there, and in order to have such privileges, you must have some position on the staff. The degree of commitment these privileges entail can range from that of pure "courtesy privileges," whereby you are responsible only for your own patients, and have nothing to do with anything else, through part-time teaching and perhaps clinic work, up to being a geographical full-time person (in which case your private load would be much smaller). To get these privileges at a big city hospital or medical center, you must be at the very least board-eligible in your specialty. The reason hospitals screen people even for courtesy privileges this way is

This obstetrician/gynecologist provides one-to-one, long-term care for her patients in private practice. She also maintains institutional connections by working in a metropolitan hospital where she is kept up-to-date with new developments in her field.

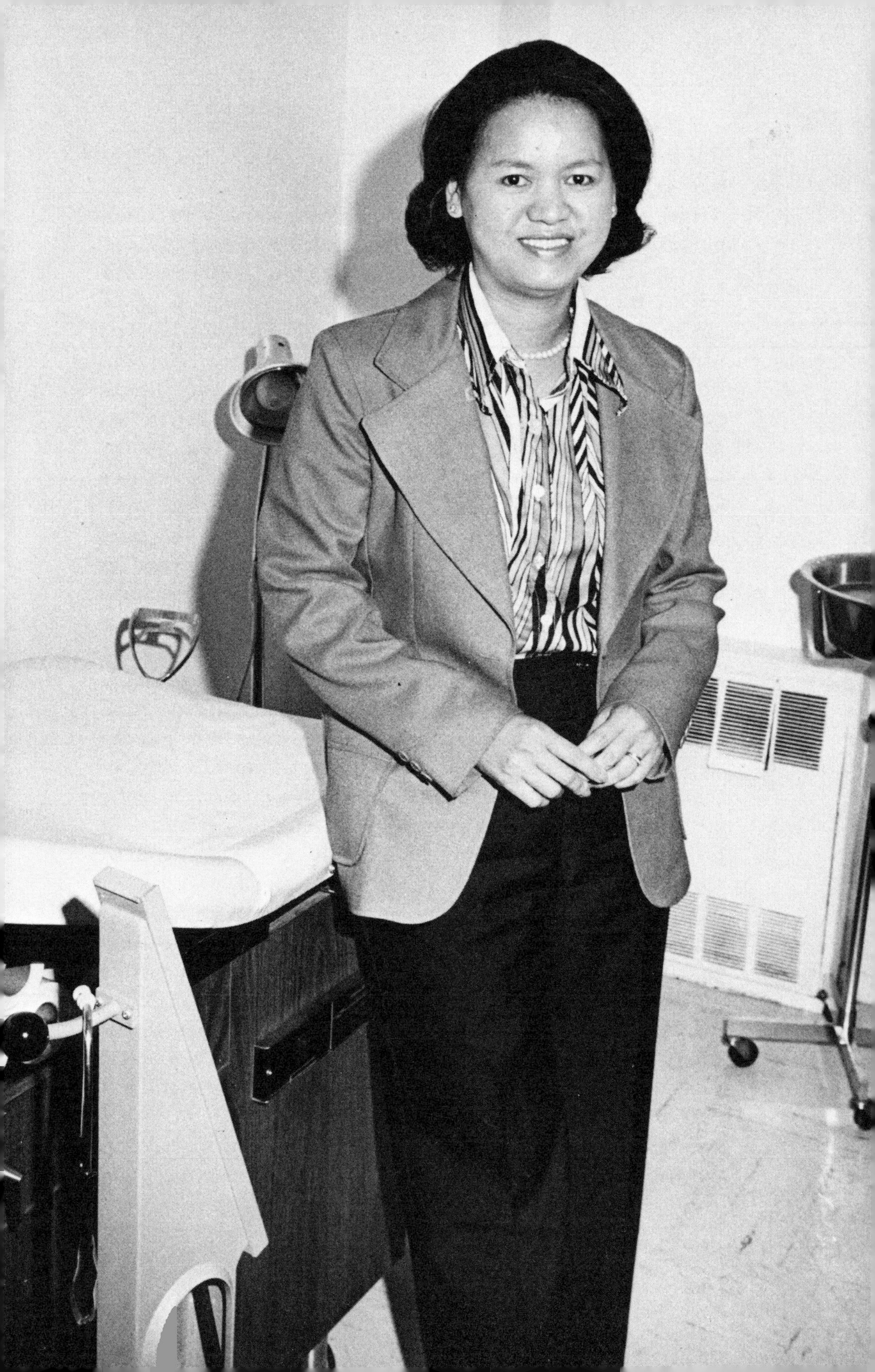

that they want to know they control the quality of the patient care going on in their wards.

The other reason for maintaining a connection with a hospital is the intellectual stimulation afforded by seeing interesting cases and talking to colleagues about them. As one woman put it, "It's the way we keep up our graduate education." Doctors in private practice do not as a rule see that many patients with difficult, complex problems, and it is these cases, the ones which require the most sophisticated diagnostic and clinical skills, that any physician regards as the true test of her professional mettle. Teaching fulfills the same function. One woman who rejected the idea of working full-time on a medical school faculty was nevertheless glad of the opportunity she had to instruct residents in her specialty twice a week, because "it's good for me to have this exposure to people who are interested in what interests me. In turn, their questions expose my field to me all over again."

One thing a number of physicians say they like about private practice is its independence and flexibility. No service chief is looking over your shoulder, and the satisfaction you have from a successful case is all your own. Also, in theory at least, you can set your own hours. (If you are in pediatrics or OBGYN, of course, your patients will set some of them for you, frequently at three o'clock in the morning.) If you elect a specialty with little or no emergency work, you actually can decide for yourself when you will be in your office. One woman who worked five days a week in a clinic and set up office hours on Saturday felt this to be the chief advantage of private practice: she could establish the work pattern that suited her needs. Most private physicians, however, seem to feel that they are at the mercy of their schedules, and that is why the majority of women choose institutional work instead of private practice. For one thing, you have to invest a certain amount of time in your practice just to keep it alive. If you don't take the time to see a certain critical mass of patients, you won't generate enough patient referrals from them, and your practice will evaporate. On the other hand, your practice may grow so large that you won't be able to find sufficient time to handle it. As one woman remarked, "It's hard to say 'no' to your first referral from a highly respected colleague, even when your forty hours are already packed." This situation has driven more than one woman back to the regular hours of hospital work.

Do not get the idea, however, that you will be besieged by an army of patients the minute you leave your residency. Most private physicians, when they begin practice, and especially specialists, find the situation to be just the reverse. They have to wait for other doctors to refer patients to them, and sometimes they wait a long time. If you begin your practice in the same geographical area that you worked or studied in before, you may have the advantage of nearby colleagues who know you. If you are relocating, however, the problem is aggravated. One psychiatrist in this situation finally put her name in the Yellow Pages ("a locally accepted practice," she explained in the AMWA's *Career Choices for Women in Medicine,* even though doctors are not allowed to advertise in the usual sense of the word), and that helped her get more patients from the area. She also had another source for referrals, one which would not be of much use to other physicians: the local minister, who would call her "when he could see he was getting in over his head."

Once physicians' referrals have equipped you with a loyal body of patients, they themselves will start sending people to you. At this point you can finally say that you have a successful medical practice. The whole process can take such a long time, though, that one woman stated that she probably could not have survived financially if she had not had a husband to support her.

There is, however, a bright side to this problem: a woman can turn that lean period into an advantage by using it to start her family. One surgeon recalled how her service chief had told her she absolutely could not continue in her residency if she became pregnant, and she thinks he was right. "I was on my feet

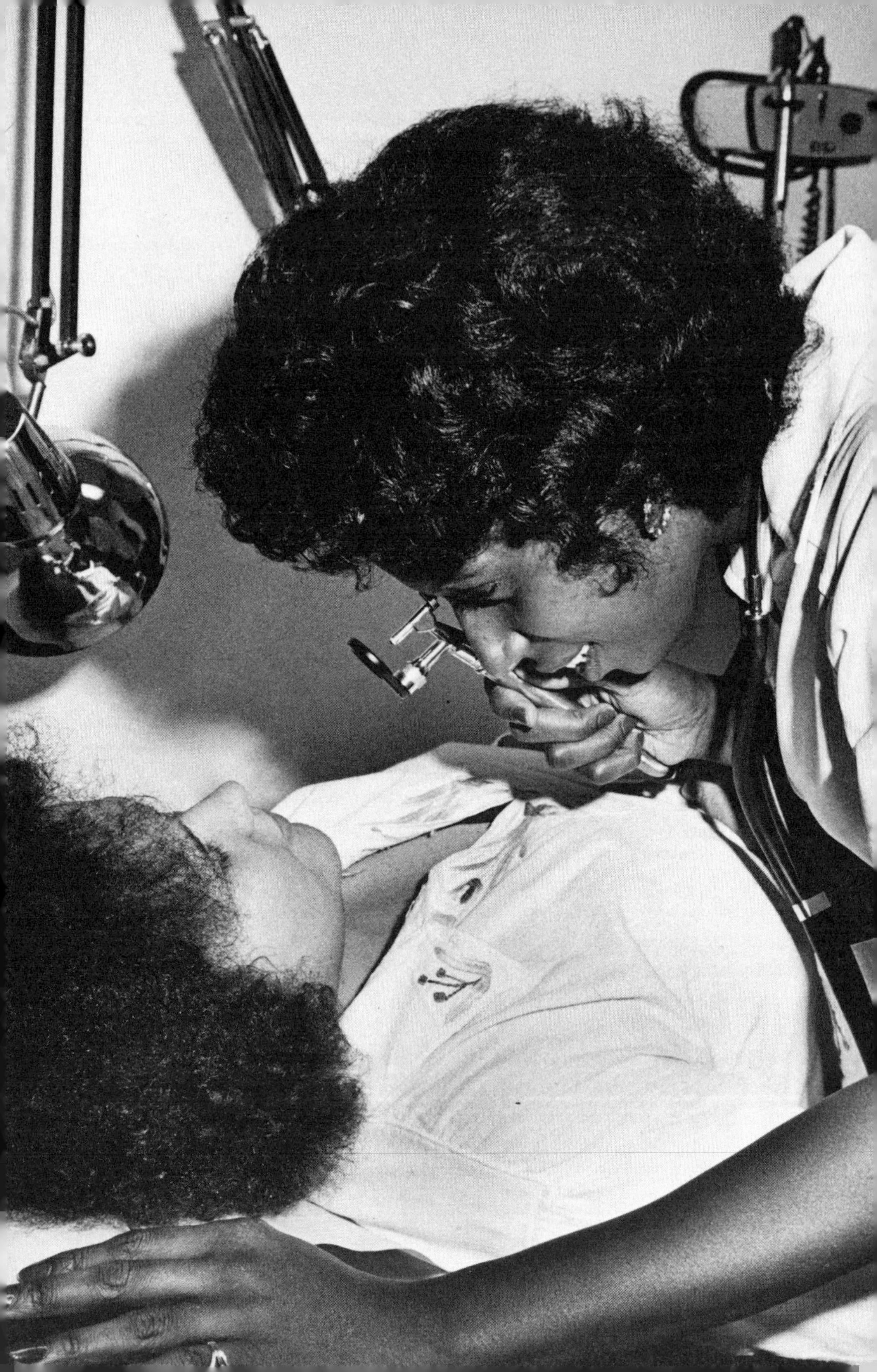

eight hours a day then," she said, "and it would have been *absolutely impossible.* I waited until I was out and had opened an office. I had almost no patients those first few years, and I was able to be a full-time mother without ever calling an official halt to my career." If your office is located in your apartment or home, you will have an ideal setting for combining a new family with a fledgling practice. The psychiatrist mentioned above had a small son who was proud of his responsibility to play quietly by himself when his mother was talking to a patient, and whose sandbox doubled as equipment for her young patients' play therapy.

But practices, even if they do take a while to grow, reach full size long before children do, and the woman in her own office is left with the question of how to cope with the responsibilities of both. One possible solution is something called "group practice." A group can consist of two or three physicians in the same specialty—also called a partnership—or a slightly larger number of practitioners representing a variety of specialties. A group can also be a small number of doctors in a given specialty from the same hospital who want to "go private" in order to handle the referrals they are getting and to take care of their patients' follow-ups. In such a case their office will usually be either very near the hospital or actually in the faculty practice area of the hospital. These doctors may work on a fee-for-service basis, each being paid by her own patients, or they may pool their earnings and share them according to the amount of time put in. The one thing all groups have in common is that the doctors share the same office, equipment, and assistants.

Two doctors sharing an office is not a particularly new idea. The distinctive feature of group work is that the doctors going

It took several years for this general practitioner to build the thriving private practice she enjoys today.

into it agree there will be some professional flow between them, and that they will be ready to accept a certain amount of responsibility for each other's patients when necessary. It is the latter feature which causes many women who have tried both ways to believe that this is the *only* way a woman could ever practice privately.

"Solo practice is impossible," one flatly stated. "The demands on me just became too great. I felt I had a responsibility to my family, but I also knew my patients had nowhere else to go when they needed me. Starting my partnership made life possible for me all over again. Now I can transfer my cases to my partner if something comes up, and know they'll be well taken care of." Of course, it will be easiest for you to use the group setting as a backup if your co-workers are in your own specialty, but even in a mixed group you will at least know, as will your patients, that *someone will always be there*. Additionally, if you are in a mixed group and have to make a referral, you and your patient will be happier if the other specialist is on the premises. (Some doctors, however, say that this limits them too much, since they feel obligated to refer only within the group.) One of the biggest advantages of any kind of group practice lies in the financial savings realized. Office rental, medical equipment, and the salaries paid to receptionists, nurses, and assistants are all very high these days. Rent alone might take 50 to 60 percent of your income, one doctor warned. When two or more physicians share these goods and services, it costs each only a fraction of what it might be otherwise.

However, there is one business expense each physician must meet on her own, group or no group, and that's the cost of malpractice insurance. The expense of this is enormous and is increasing all the time. Surgeons are the hardest hit of all—as of this writing, they must pay a yearly minimum of approximately $20,000 in insurance premiums, and neurosurgeons may pay as much as $30,000. The specialties with the lowest rates are psychiatry and pediatrics: their premiums cost about $2,000 a year.

For the most part, these skyrocketing rates reflect the fact that more people are, indeed, taking their doctors to court. According to an article in *Science News* (May 26, 1973), 14,500 claims were filed in 1970, and statisticians estimated that by 1975 the number would rise to approximately 20,000. The vast majority of these claims are settled out of court, primarily because court costs are so high that many physicians are willing to pay a few thousand dollars to avoid them, even though the legal odds may be slightly in their favor. Of the cases that did go to court in 1970, says *Science News,* 54 percent were decided for the physicians.

What is it that makes so many patients sue? I personally suspect that a lot of people in this country became aware of their litigative options at the same time that they became convinced that medical technology could do anything. People are daily bombarded with news of the incredible strides science is making: organ transplants, open-heart surgery, and the like. If doctors can do all these things, yet sometimes can't set a fracture correctly or use a needle without hitting a nerve, then people are apt to feel betrayed. In the old days, when typically a doctor was a family friend who had delivered the children and their mothers before them, people naturally were much more hesitant about taking legal action. Nowadays the physician is more typically a specialist in a big hospital, someone the patient and family saw only once. They feel differently about her, especially when they see how much she is charging them. The high cost and impersonality of much medical care today, coupled with the popular assumption that all physicians enjoy a luxurious lifestyle, have caused many people to resent the medical profession. The medical profession has always had its detractors, but this attitude has become something more of a social phenomenon in recent years.

There is an additional element contributing to the fact that insurance companies which specialize in malpractice coverage have found it necessary to charge doctors so much. As high as premiums are, they still do not cover the cost of all the cases that arise. To make up the difference, insurance companies invest heavily in the stock market. When the market took a sudden dive a few years ago, one company had to triple its premiums all over the country. Anesthesiologists in California, who had to increase their yearly payments from $5,000 to $18,000 in one month, revolted and went on strike on May 1, 1975. Many doctors feel that a physician's commitment to her patients precludes this sort of action, but they agree that it is manifestly unfair that doctors should be so heavily penalized for something that is not even a medical problem, in no way reflecting their own professional performance.

The cost of malpractice insurance has caused many doctors to leave private practice, even though private practitioners make more money than any other kind of physician, and some make more than almost anybody at all. In addition, the demands of private practice, both as regards time and commitment, have caused increasing numbers of physicians—men and women alike—to decide against it in recent years. Some students of the situation say that, as a result, the face of medical care in this country is changing, slowly but perceptibly. Nevertheless, private practice is still a long way from becoming a thing of the past. There will always be doctors for whom the practice of medicine means first of all ministering to people directly and on their own, doctors who agree with the woman who said, "You're really missing something—and I think it's the biggest thing—if you don't have that warm, personal relationship at the basis of your work."

7

Public Health

Do you like to work with other people at solving problems, the bigger and trickier they are, the better? Do you enjoy finding out about the way things are done in order to find ways to get them done better? In short, do you like to try to make things happen? If you do, you will probably be attracted to public health, the most political way of practicing medicine.

There is probably no other field of medical practice in which the job possibilities are so numerous and varied. Here is a small sampling of the things you could do: You could direct a planned parenthood clinic. You could work for a state agency engaged in research for planning the administration of health care. You could give patients instruction in self-care at a local outpatient clinic. You could teach preventive medicine in medical school. You could run a satellite clinic for a public hospital in an inner-city neighborhood. You could work on a statewide fluoridation program with a team of local doctors and dentists. You could do federally funded research in a storefront setting on the interrelation of health and environment. You could be the medical liaison for a group of voluntary agencies trying to set up a statewide geriatric program. Or you could go live in

Paris and work for the United States Public Health Service Quarantine Program, reviewing the records of people wishing to enter the United States.

The framework into which these and hundreds more jobs fit sprawls across the country and extends from the federal level down to the smallest communities. It is in the latter, at the local level, that you would find the most opportunity for work involving direct patient contact. In New York City, whose public health system has become the model for most large cities in the country and is studied by public health workers from all over the world, there are about sixteen such district centers, maintaining programs for VD, TB, sickle cell anemia, drug addiction, prenatal care, pediatrics, dentistry, and so on. There is also a system of public hospitals run by the Health and Hospitals Corporation.

On the state level, most of the work involves setting up and supervising local programs, training personnel, organizing epidemiological research, and studying zoonotic problems (diseases transmitted to human being by animals). There is some direct patient work available here, because states will occasionally send out physicians to work in underserved areas, but most of the jobs are administrative and organizational.

At the federal level, under the aegis of the Department of Health, Education and Welfare, there is the United States Public Health Service itself. The PHS has three sub-agencies: the NIH, the Consumer Protection and Environmental Health Agency, and the Health Services and Mental Health Administration. The NIH has already been discussed. The second agency deals with air pollution, water supply problems, drug, food, and product safety, solid waste disposal, and so forth. The third is divided into a number of smaller agencies dealing with the administration of health care. It is through this agency that money, services, and technical assistance are filtered down to the local level.

Finally, there are voluntary agencies, not connected with the government. These are private, non-profit organizations devoted to funding and programming research into health problems, usually the cures of serious diseases. The best known are the big ones, such as the American Heart Association and the American Cancer Society, but there are at least 20,000 more of varying sizes.

To enter the field of public health, you have to earn the degree of Master of Public Health (MPH) at one of the twenty or so public health schools currently in existence. At one time you had to have an M.D. degree before you could attend these schools, but they now admit people from other health professions, with less advanced degrees, reflecting the fact that public health has expanded to include statistical and administrative as well as medical work. A doctorate in public health is also available, and is taken chiefly by people who plan to teach. Physicians who pursue a degree in public health usually have completed their residencies in a specialty, although it is also possible to take a residency in preventive medicine or public health itself, for example at one of the nation's eleven federally run hospitals. Examinations for certification in public health are given by the American Board of Preventive Medicine.

You can get a good idea of what public health physicians actually do by considering the major courses of study offered by public health schools. For example, there is *biostatistics.* This course concerns the collection, ordering, and analysis of data about health problems. No research can be done until statistics have proved that there is something going on that cannot be attributed to chance alone. You have to be *very* interested in and good at math in order to go into this field—a background in calculus is recommended. The people who do go into it are often not doctors, but they *are* often women because the hours are probably the most regular in the whole medical field.

Epidemiology is detective work on the causes of disease. The following is a sample case: A few years ago, a Boston physician was astonished to find a number of very young women coming to him—all within a relatively short time—each exhibiting an extremely rare type of vaginal cancer. Since this particular form of the disease has traditionally turned up only once in twenty years, it was clear that something was going on. After an exhaustive study of the patients' histories, it was finally discovered that their mothers had all taken a certain drug during their pregnancies. It had not affected the male fetuses in any way, but it caused this cancer in all the females—a cancer which did not become apparent until fifteen or twenty years after the girls were born. "Clusters of very rare cases in time and space—that's what we immediately go after," an epidemiologist explained. "The very common cancers, like breast and uterus, are the ones it's hardest to find the cause for, because it could be anything. To make epidemiology work, you need a very good clinician—I mean one who's alert to everything he sees—and an epidemiologist who will know how to investigate what he's found." As its name suggests, epidemiology used to be concerned only with infectious diseases. As more of these yielded to vaccines and improved sanitation measures, and as it became apparent that it was possible to find causes for things like cancer (the discovery of the link to smoking was instrumental in this), epidemiologists turned their attention to the causes and distribution of human diseases in general.

They can often be found working hand in hand with physicians in *environmental science,* who study the technical end of pollution problems in such areas as air, water, solid wastes, and radiation and pest control. A lot of laboratory work is involved in environmental science, and a background in chemistry or biochemistry is called for. A private practitioner may find a certain gastrointestinal complaint recurring in her patients. She will contact an epidemiologist, who will be able to locate the source of the problem, perhaps in the water supply. Then an environmental scientist will work on finding out what is in the water supply to cause the sickness, and how it got there in the first place. Finally, a public health official will take whatever steps are necessary to keep the harmful element out of the water in the future.

Community psychiatry is another field of public health work. You might assume that the problems dealt with by psychiatrists are too personal and individual to be appropriately treated in a public context, but there is a way in which the two connect. As one woman put it, "Community psychiatry is like a link between individual psychiatry and epidemiology. A G.P. [general practicianer] will treat people suffering from food poisoning after a church supper, but an epidemiologist will look for the cause. Well, we look at the psychological problems which recur in a population the same way. We say, 'What are the risk factors here; what's going on? Let's see, these are all middle-aged women who had their first babies late in life.' " Group therapy was originally a public health concept, because community psychiatrists found it the most efficient way of working with this kind of problem, although they readily admit that not everyone can be treated that way.

If you want to go into public health in order to change the way things are done, because you believe they could be done much better, then go into *medical care administration,* which has been described by one practitioner as the attempt "to bring the peaks of medical care to the valleys which have never seen it." "You are needed," she went on, "by the multitude of patients who have fallen through the cracks in our present medical care system." Medical care administration is for the woman who is willing to forgo patient contact in favor of helping to solve the social, administrative, economic, and political problems which allow these cracks to exist. The background needed in this field is not a scientific discipline like math or chemistry, but a wide ranging familiarity with the medical field, politics, and people. You will have to know about hospital administration, health insurance, city finances, legislative processes, bookkeeping, and bureaucracy. ("Bureaucracy" is perhaps the word most frequently on the lips of anyone who has ever worked in public health, with "innovation" a close second—the two being understood to be in a sort of adversary relationship.)

One of the central concepts of public health is that there are aspects of health and illness which cannot be dealt with simply through the contact between the individual patient and doctor. Thus, while medical care administration searches the institutional superstructure for the causes of inadequate care, *socio-medical science* (often called *social* or *community medicine*) is looking for the underlying sources of medical problems, typically in the patient's environment. These can be drug abuse, inadequate nutrition, faulty sanitary facilities, lead in the paint on the walls, etc. "You can go to a medicaid center and they'll lay on hands right away," one professor commented. "That's no answer. They'll do something about a patient's rheumatism, maybe, but they won't, they can't, do anything about the oozing walls of the tenement he lives in. Then he'll go straight back to them and get sick all over again. As long as we don't address ourselves to things like those walls, we're not doing anything about the problem."

Public health has always attracted large numbers of women. In fact, school health and family planning services have been dominated by them from the beginning. Ask anyone "why," and the answer probably will be "The hours!" It is true that clinical or administrative work will not keep you away from home at night, or call you out on emergencies. (It is also true that clinic work doesn't pay terribly well, but a woman with a working husband is often free not to worry so much about her salary.) Still, hours are not the only explanation. Most women involved in public health express a sense of social commitment to the

This former nurse, director of nursing, air force major, and project director for the Urban League, brings a wealth of experience to her current job as an administrator for Planned Parenthood. She provides consulting services and technical assistance to the organization's 189 affiliates located in 43 states and the District of Columbia. Her work eventually will enable thousands of people to control their own lives.

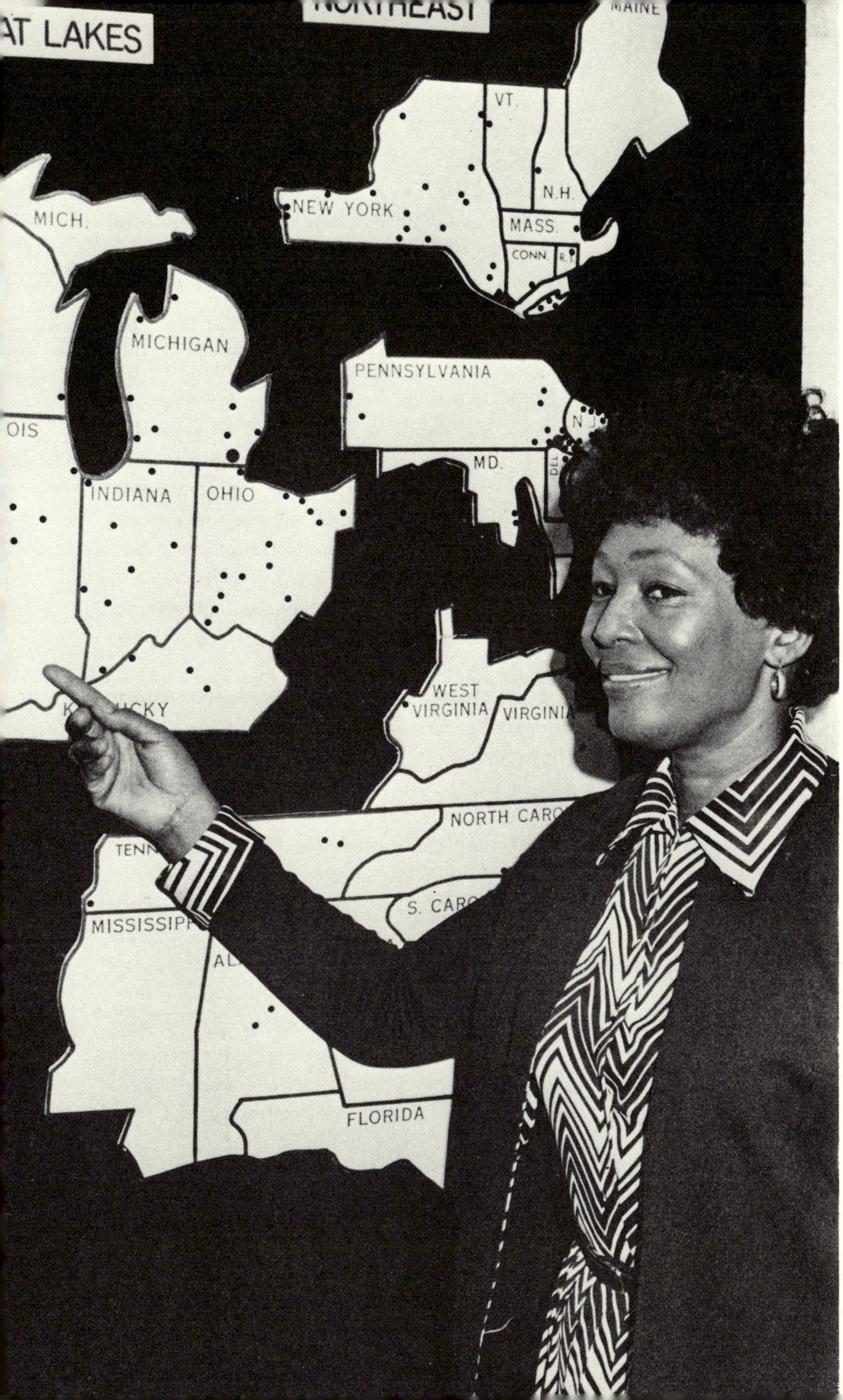
MAINE
VT.
N.H.
NEW YORK
MASS.
CONN.
MICH.
MICHIGAN
PENNSYLVANIA
MD.
INDIANA
OHIO
WEST VIRGINIA
VIRGINIA
FLORIDA

work they are doing. One even said, "I liked the idea of administration and politics. I'm a glutton for aggravation!" The most important factor, however, may be that one of the largest components of public health work is pediatrics, and more women go into pediatrics than into any other specialty. The New York City system includes prenatal clinics, maternal-child health centers, well-baby clinics (for routine monthly check-ups), and pediatric treatment centers for sick children, and many of the doctors working in these centers are women. "I think women are extremely well equipped to handle maternal and child health, and not just because of their 'instincts,' " one woman said. "When I was in well-baby work in the slums of New Haven, in 98 percent of the cases the baby was fine, but the mother was upset because she was so exhausted! That's far more important. A woman would understand that. Also, a woman opens up to another woman. A man might tell her she had to rinse the diapers three times—with three kids and another on the way!"

Sharon works in a well-baby clinic in a black and Hispanic neighborhood, and describes her work this way: "I see the indigent patients. They seem pleased at what goes on here. They don't follow the lists of instructions as slavishly as middle-class women. They think the doctor has some kind of magic shot somewhere and I think they come more for that than for the advice they get." Sharon doesn't envision herself making much of an impact in alleviating community ills. What she likes about her clinic is that it provides something similar to a private practice setting for people who could not afford to have one otherwise. At the same time, she feels that working in the public sector necessarily imposes certain restraints on her. "I have no control over my patients after they leave me," she explained. "In a private practice situation I could refer a patient to a doctor I know and respect, who knows and respects me. I used to send many more patients to our affiliated hospital in the days when I still knew the house staff and I could call up someone I knew and explain the situation."

Women in public health are not only to be found working with other women and children, however. There are plenty of them behind administrative desks. "I have no patients of my own any more, but I don't feel too deprived," says one such woman in the New York City system. "We're doing something very important here. Our goal is to set standards and determine the level that constitutes good care in the city's hospitals. We don't do it sitting in an ivory tower. We work with service chiefs, county medical societies, and the Greater New York Hospital Association. We try to get Blue Cross and Medicaid to say they won't pay a hospital unless it meets certain standards. And we keep our eyes open. For instance, a few years ago a warning was issued to hospitals when it was discovered that certain oxygen equipment constituted a threat with regard to congenital blindness. They hadn't been careless, they just hadn't known."

It is not always that easy, of course. One doctor doing abortions after they became legal in 1973 was in the habit of sending his patients home to await developments once he had injected the saline solution that killed the fetus. "I had to explain to him that that wasn't the way it was done," this woman remembered with a shudder. "I try not to make enemies, but sometimes it's unavoidable. Sometimes, they try to get back at you, but it doesn't really matter. More important things are at stake here."

It is true that one of the most important requirements for public health work is an ability to deal with people. Another kind of interpersonal hassle was reported by Helen as one of her biggest professional headaches. She is a dentist who runs an outpatient clinic in lower Manhattan, serving a neighborhood that includes black, Puerto Rican, Italian, and Chinese families. "The hospital of which we're a satellite sends droves of people over here to sit in my office whenever I have to fire a paraprofessional," she said. "They're terrified of community pressure over there, and immediately take on anyone I have to let go. It is required by law that all our paras have to live in the neighborhood—they're our interpreters—and plenty of them are fine, but some aren't. There was one girl who always came late or wouldn't show up at all. And she hated the patients! She'd curse them out to their faces. Others can't come in sometimes because they have too many problems at home. I'm not running a welfare center for them, I'm trying to provide services." Helen hasn't had to reprimand any doctors or dentists, but if she did "I'd just write them a very terse note. You're dealing with a different population there."

Helen is pleased with the job she has done with the clinic, increasing the number of pediatricians working there from one to three, setting up a full-time three-chair dental clinic, and introducing services in ophthalmology, audiology, and family planning. In fact, she feels there is virtually nothing left for her to do there, and it is partly for that reason that she is thinking of going back to teaching. But the real reason she would like to leave is that, like everyone else working for the city of New York, she is in constant fear of having her funds cut off. "I never know from one day to the next when the city is going to terminate this place," she said. "I'd probably stay on, if only there weren't that uncertainty."

In public health work there is uncertainty and there are money problems; there is bureaucracy and inefficiency. There is a tremendous amount that needs to be learned, and still more that needs to be done. And there is an almost infinite number of ways you can select from to help do it—if you are so inclined, and if you think you have the special energy and hardy optimism called for by public health work.

8

Occupational Medicine

If you think you would like to practice in a setting that would combine the kind of patient contact you could have in a small community with regular hours and a steady income, you might think about occupational medicine, which is concerned with taking care of the health of all the workers in a given factory or company. (It has nothing to do with occupational therapy, or physical therapy.) It used to be called industrial medicine, and that term lingers on in common usage, but it is somewhat misleading since it suggests that the field is concerned only with the health problems of workers in factories or heavy industry—what is called "plant medicine." Most large corporations now have programs set up at their own expense to safeguard the health of their office workers as well. Smaller companies usually have some such arrangement too—depending on the size of the work force, it can be as modest as a single nurse in an office. In such a case, the company may reserve a part of the daily hours of a nearby private physician and send workers to his office when they need more care than the nurse can provide. Of course, companies like IBM, American Telephone and Telegraph, J. C. Penney, Exxon, and Union Carbide, with their thousands of employees, boast medical programs of considerable scope and sophistication.

Insurance companies were among the first to set up these office health programs, precisely because their work gives them a keener sense of the uncertainties of life. Some of their programs are considered among the best in the country. A woman who works in one said earnestly, "I work here with pride. This company has been known for years for its fine department. We are the personal physicians for five thousand people, the front line of the whole medical profession for them. We find cancer, we find heart trouble, we find diabetes and hypertension. We have our own lab; I can give blood pressure and blood sugar tests when they're necessary. If someone has a heart problem, we could go a few steps down the hall for an electrocardiogram and I could have a special heart attack ambulance over here in three minutes. And we have a beautiful physical therapy department upstairs. No private practitioner could possibly have all those facilities."

Another source of pleasure for this woman was the personal element in her work. "Most of our people have worked here for years—we get to know their whole lives. It's more like working in the town of 7,000 where I grew up than my private practice in the middle of Manhattan!" Like the general practitioner, the office physician is dealing with a fairly stable, healthy, and continuing population which is limited to the members of a single community. And, like the G.P., she will be making referrals to specialists whenever something out of the ordinary comes up. This is true because, although many company programs have sophisticated diagnostic equipment and the facilities for dealing with on-the-spot emergencies, their doctors do not do the actual long-term treatment for serious cases. After a worker's heart condition or ulcer has been diagnosed, he will be referred to a cardiologist or gastroenterologist on the outside whom the company has retained for such work. In keeping with this role of being on the "front line" of medical treatment, most occupational physicians are in internal medicine or general practice, as opposed to the narrower specialties.

Of course, not every physician would find attractive the relative predictability of this kind of practice. One woman in charge of an occupational program regretted that she could not attract many young doctors because most of the cases were not very challenging. This lack of challenge leads some physicians to regard occupational medicine as less intellectually demanding than other fields. "You have to have a strong ego to go into occupational medicine," one woman remarked. "We're at the bottom of the prestige totem pole."

Nevertheless, it is not true that the occupational physician in an office setting does nothing but wait around for people to come in for a check-up or have a heart attack. Enterprising women in charge of such programs have set up smoke-ending clinics, obesity clinics, self-help groups for alcoholics, and other beneficial projects for the workers they serve. One woman in charge of employee health at a hospital where the patients are nearly all terminal cancer cases observed the effects of this work on the staff—she called it "the Memorial syndrome"—and set up a psychiatric self-help program for them. "It helps them to give better care by understanding themselves better," she explained. "Their patients die, and it causes them terrific feelings of anger, frustration, hopelessness, and grief. They take it out on others, and themselves too. I've been trying to get an in-service program in transactional analysis and Gestalt therapy added on."

Employees working in close proximity to death aren't the only ones likely to need more than physical healing from their company doctors. One occupational physician who had the experience of a year of psychiatric residency said she found it a definite advantage in her work. "You hear much more about emotional problems than another kind of doctor might," she said. "People come in with problems about the stresses and strains of their jobs, about their relationships with their fellow

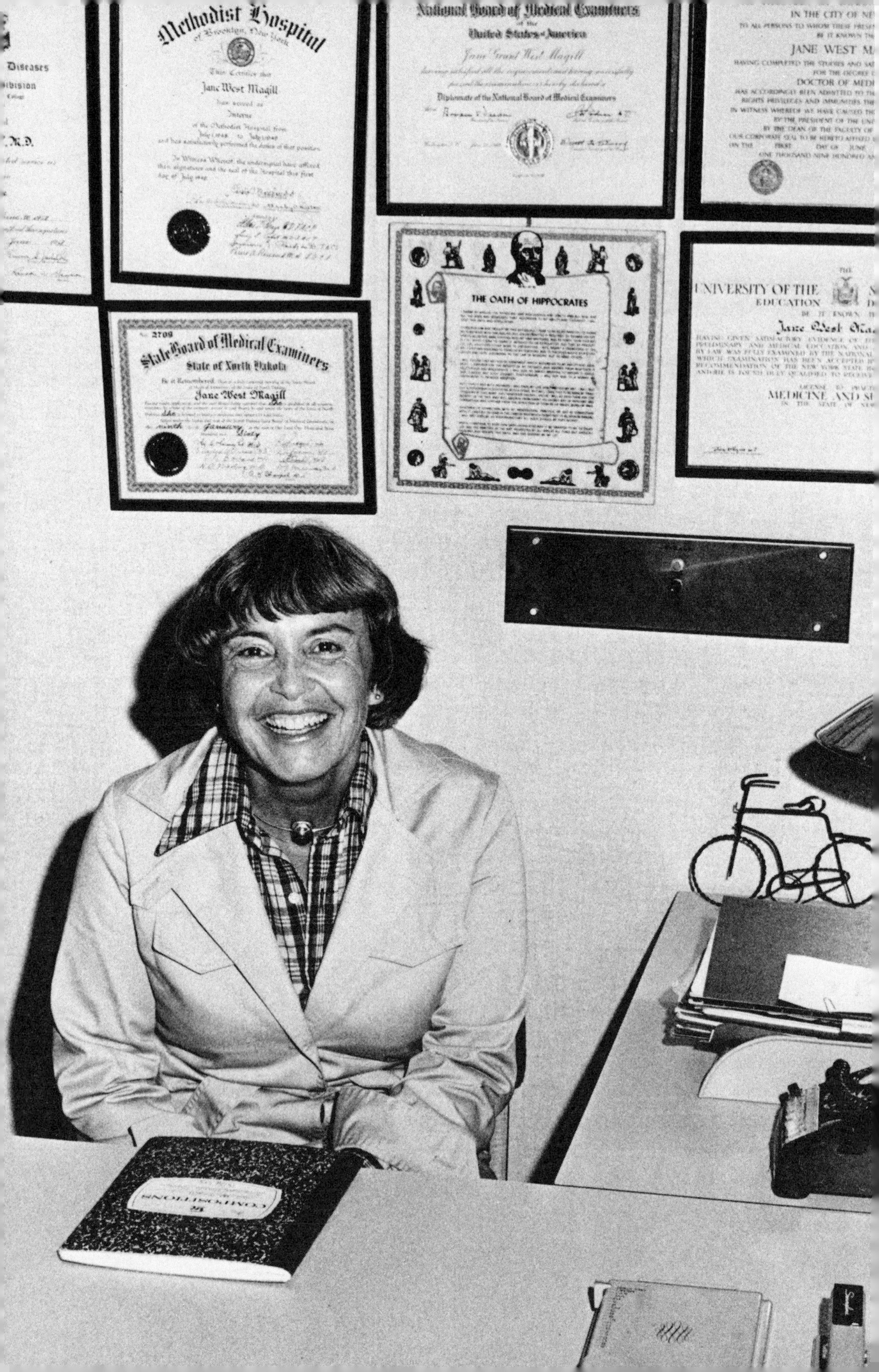
Methodist Hospital
of Brooklyn, New York
Jane West Magill
National Board of Medical Examiners
United States of America
Jane Grant West Magill
Diplomate of the National Board of Medical Examiners
JANE WEST M
DOCTOR OF MED
THE OATH OF HIPPOCRATES
2709
State Board of Medical Examiners
State of North Dakota
Jane West Magill
UNIVERSITY OF THE
EDUCATION
Jane West Ma
MEDICINE AND S
COMPOSITIONS

workers and their families." It is probably true that a patient will feel it more appropriate to talk to the doctor about such problems when his or her medical care is being administered in the context of employment. The doctor's office is usually physically on the business premises, and the employee knows the company put it there.

An additional aspect of this kind of program which should be mentioned is that many of the jobs it offers are part-time. The advantages of this are obvious for a woman who, for example, wants to be home every day at three o'clock when her children get out of school. Occupational medicine is, in fact, an excellent choice if you want to maintain a low professional profile for a while. You will never have to rush to the hospital during the weekend to check on a patient in intensive care, or to the lab to note the progress of a culture. Also, if you are interested in setting up a private practice, but are concerned about the scarcity of patients and referrals during the first few years, and the financial insecurity that entails, a part-time job in occupational medicine can help to take up the slack. The salaries are not the highest in the medical world, but they can form a cushion until your practice begins to pay. Then you can follow the example of the woman who gradually decreased the number of hours a week she committed to the company as the number of her patients grew, until she had made a complete changeover.

This doctor directs the employee health program at a hospital where most of the patients are terminal cancer cases. Dealing with death often produces extreme stress. It is the job of occupational medicine to deal with the psychological hazards of a job situation as well as the physical ones.

If office medicine presents some of the features of private practice, plant medicine has a number of the characteristics of public health work. The plant physician is working with a patient population whose health problems will be determined in part by their environment, and she has to know everything medically relevant about that environment. And, like the public health physician, she has to be good at working on medical problems with non-medical people from a variety of disciplines, in this case management and labor representatives, safety engineers or industrial hygienists, state inspectors, lawyers, social workers, etc.

The plant physician makes sure that the worker is fit for the job and that the plant is fit for the workers. Are the walkways clear of machines with dangerous moving parts? What kinds of particles or fumes are generated in the course of the work, and are there provisions for dealing with them? Are there machines which give off contaminating substances, and, if so, are there hoods to siphon them off, and are these near the exhaust vents? These questions and others are tackled by the plant physician, working in conjunction with the industrial hygienist, who takes care of the technical end and is involved in arranging the machinery. In addition, the workers may need special protective clothing: masks, goggles, earplugs. (Factories are extremely noisy places, and noise can be noxious if one is exposed to it for years on end.)

Another feature of occupational medicine is that the physician's patients and employer are two distinct parties whose interests are often believed to be in conflict. Many workers, for example, are afraid that their medical records could become instruments of job discrimination if placed in the hands of management. The Coal Mine Health and Safety Act of 1969 reflected this fear by ruling that the company physician *could not know* the results of lung X rays given to the workers, because the union was afraid there would be a rush to fire anyone suffering from lung disease. The assumption here was that the plant doctor was an agent of the company. Commenting on this, one physician suggested that plant doctors should "exteriorize" their practice, moving it out of the factory and into separate offices, to dramatize the fact that they are not instruments of the company, the union, the government, or anyone other than the sound practice of medicine itself.

But if some workers are afraid the company doctor might endanger their jobs by doing too much, other people are afraid she might risk their lives by doing too little, again at the behest of the company. A few years ago it was discovered that a number of factory workers who were exposed to vinyl chloride or asbestos were getting cancer as a result, and were dying lingering deaths. Public opinion tended to regard the management involved as indifferent to their workers' health when it conflicted with their quest for profits, possibly even to the extent of obstructing investigations which would have revealed the cause of the disease. It would be naive to try to make a blanket statement one way or the other, but you should know that a conscientious physician is not automatically or necessarily placed in such cases in an adversary relationship with her employer, as this doctor's words show:

> "One has gotten the impression that companies are more interested in money than health. I've worked for two and in each case I can truly say that the employers had the health of their workers at heart. If I ever found anything dangerous, I'd call the industrial hygienist and it would be taken care of. I think occupational medicine may be easiest in a plant, because the doctor has that kind of power. I think this is true of most of the big companies. After all, they care enough to hire doctors!"

You can become board-certified in occupational medicine by fulfilling the same kind of examination and practice requirements demanded by the medical specialty boards. The examination is given by the American Board of Preventive Medicine. There are not very many women certified in this area as of now, but there is no reason why there shouldn't be more. Occupational medicine does not offer the most exciting work in the medical world, but it is an excellent field for a woman who likes security, regularity, and people, and who wants a professional commitment that will stay within limits.

9

The Role of Nursing

Actually, this chapter has no place in this book, but you should read it anyway.

It doesn't belong here because, as any nurse will tell you, nursing is a health care profession in its own right, with its own scope and responsibilities. It is not a women's auxiliary to the medical profession, and if some people think of it that way, it is in part a result of the fact that for many years they could not imagine a physician being anything other than a man. They therefore saw nursing as the female alternative to being a doctor. During those years there were many young women who wanted to go to medical school, but were shunted into nursing instead because the people around them believed it to be more appropriate for them. Many women were bitterly frustrated as a result, and it is entirely fitting that the women's movement has attacked this syndrome by seeking to educate the public to the idea that every child has the right to try for whatever career he or she has the will and talent to pursue. At the same time, however, this should in no way be taken to mean that the demanding and vitally necessary profession of nursing should now be thrown on the scrap-heap of social history. As one R.N.

(registered nurse) tersely stated: "You will never know how hostile I become when I hear a feminist berate a woman because she's a nurse. Does liberation mean we all have to be doctors? I thought it meant being able to make choices."

Women who are asked why they made the choice of going into nursing almost always cite the same reason: wanting to help people. "I knew it was what I wanted from the time I was five, suturing my dolls," one said. "I always felt protective toward living things. I have a great concern for people's total comfort—physical as well as psychological." This characteristic is probably the first thing you should look for in yourself if you are considering nursing. A patient in a hospital may see the doctor once a day on rounds, but nurses are with the patient each hour of the day. If he or she is uncomfortable, or in pain, or despondent, or terrified, the nurses are the ones who must minister to both mind and body. The fact that they have to scrape bedsores and empty bedpans in the course of doing all this leads many people to view the nursing profession as one devoted primarily to cleaning up things. "My parents were against the idea of my becoming a nurse," one woman recalled, "because, out of innocent ignorance, they thought it was a menial and demeaning job. But I never believed that, and I don't now. I've always seen nursing as a humanistic whole."

There are three different kinds of training programs that can lead to a nursing career: the two-year associate program, the three-year diploma program, and the four-year baccalaureate program. The associate program is offered in junior and community colleges and involves very little theoretical material,

Most women who go into nursing do so because they want to help other people, in this case, infants. Nurses provide care for the whole person—physical and psychological. Here we see a pediatric nurse (left) conferring with an infant-care technician.

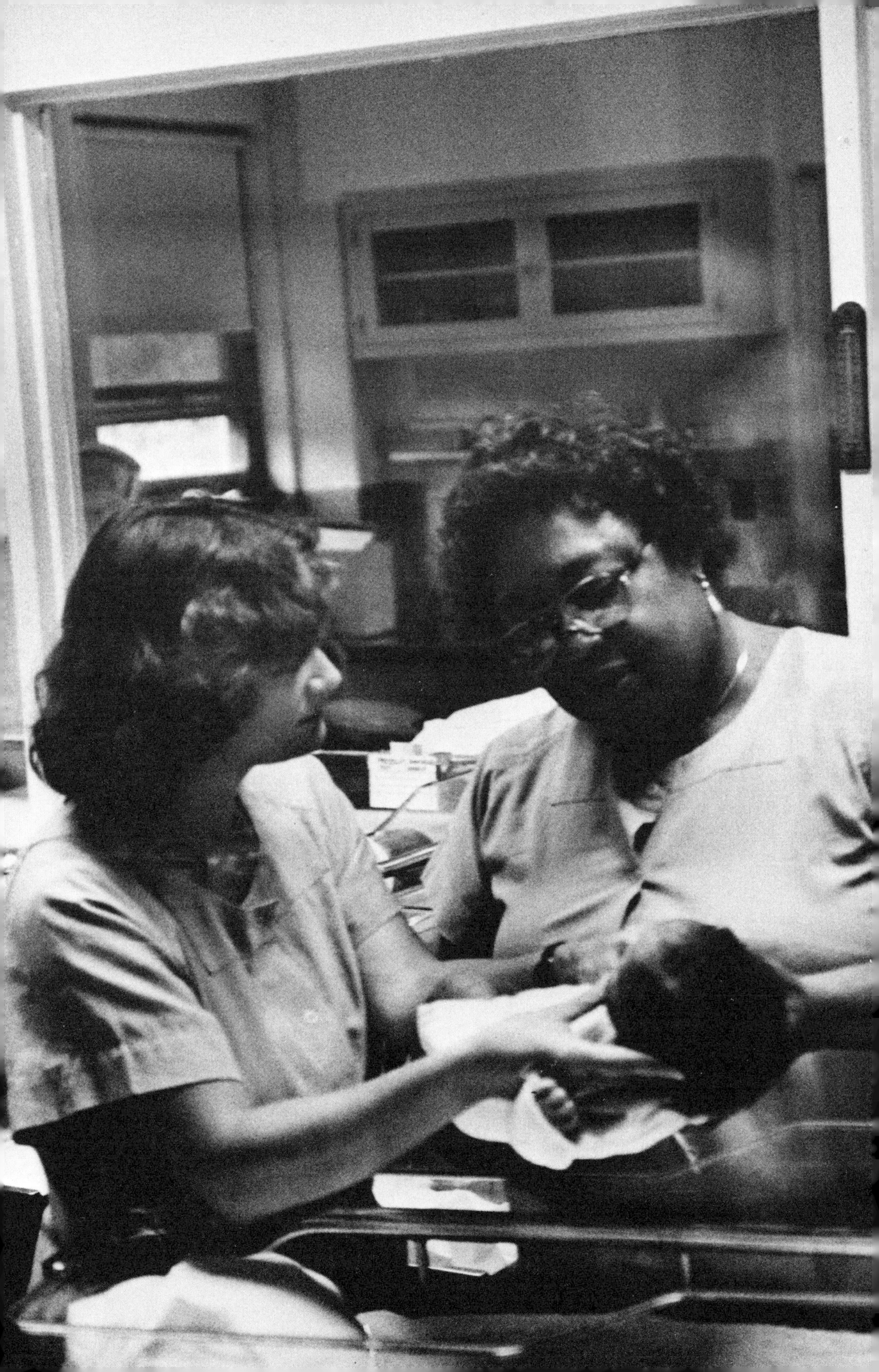

but offers the advantage of equipping a woman to work as a nurse in the shortest time possible. Diploma degrees are given by hospital schools, where much of the training is done on the wards and floors of the affiliated hospitals themselves. Nursing educators emphasize that clinical experience is by far the most important component in the training of a good nurse, and the quality of a diploma program is judged by the ease with which its graduates can make the transition from student to practicing nurse once they enter the profession.

Finally, the baccalaureate program grooms women for jobs in teaching, administration, and nursing research, the latter studying nursing techniques and investigating how to improve them. These programs are offered in colleges and universities, with the students enrolled taking a regular undergraduate liberal arts course and majoring in nursing. Some hospital-affiliated baccalaureate programs themselves require a college degree for admission.

The American Nurses' Association publishes a booklet listing all the nursing schools in the country accredited by the National League for Nursing, indicating whether they give associate, diploma, or baccalaureate programs. It is titled *Schools of Nursing: A Directory of RN Programs,* and costs 50 cents. You can get it by writing to the ANA, 2420 Pershing Road, Kansas City, Mo., 64108. It is advisable to send away for it early, so that you can then write to the schools you are interested in and find out which high school courses each requires for admission. You might also be interested in two booklets put out by the National League for Nursing, 10 Columbus Circle, New York, N.Y., 10019, which tell about financial assistance for nursing students. One is *Scholarships and Loans—Beginning Education in Nursing* (1972), publication number 41–410, and is meant for associate and diploma applicants. The other, for baccalaureate students, is called *Scholarships, Fellowships, Educational Grants and Loans for Registered Nurses* (1973), publication number 41–408. Each booklet costs 25 cents.

As you can see, the three types of training programs vary

considerably as to the kind and amount of instruction they provide. Nevertheless, all nursing graduates, whether associate, diploma, or baccalaureate, take the same state board exam for licensing after they graduate, and all get the same title, Registered Nurse, upon passing it. There is one kind of nurse, however, who is not an R.N.—an L.P.N., or licensed practical nurse. An L.P.N., whose training lasts 12 to 18 months, performs some of the less technical functions of nursing, like checking the patient's temperature, pulse, and respiration, giving blood pressure tests and alcohol rubs, applying compresses, placing catheters, and dressing wounds. A list of schools giving courses leading to a practical nurse's license can be found in the pamphlet *Practical Nursing Careers,* published by the Careers Department of the NLN. It costs 50 cents and can be ordered by mail.

Universities also confer master's and doctorate degrees in nursing which are taken primarily by baccalaureate graduates who intend to go on to teaching and the higher administrative jobs. A nurse can take a master's degree in a functional major, such as nursing service administration, or a clinical specialty, such as cardiology or oncology (cancer work). Doctoral work might be more theoretical in nature. One nurse who is now a professor in a baccalaureate program, and had always been interested in obstetrics and maternal-child care, wrote her doctoral essay on the attitudes of baccalaureate nurses toward women having elective abortions.

Diploma-trained nurses can become administrators as well (a move considered by some to be prestigious), but it means leaving patients behind, something not all of them are willing to do. Many nurses lament the fact that all of the prestige in the nursing world seems to be attached to administrative posts, while bedside care, the real backbone of the profession, is demeaned. "We need to make the practicing bedside nurse appreciated for her skills once more," one woman stated. Now a highly placed administrator in the New York City Public Health System, she says, "Today I miss patient contact. I was truly

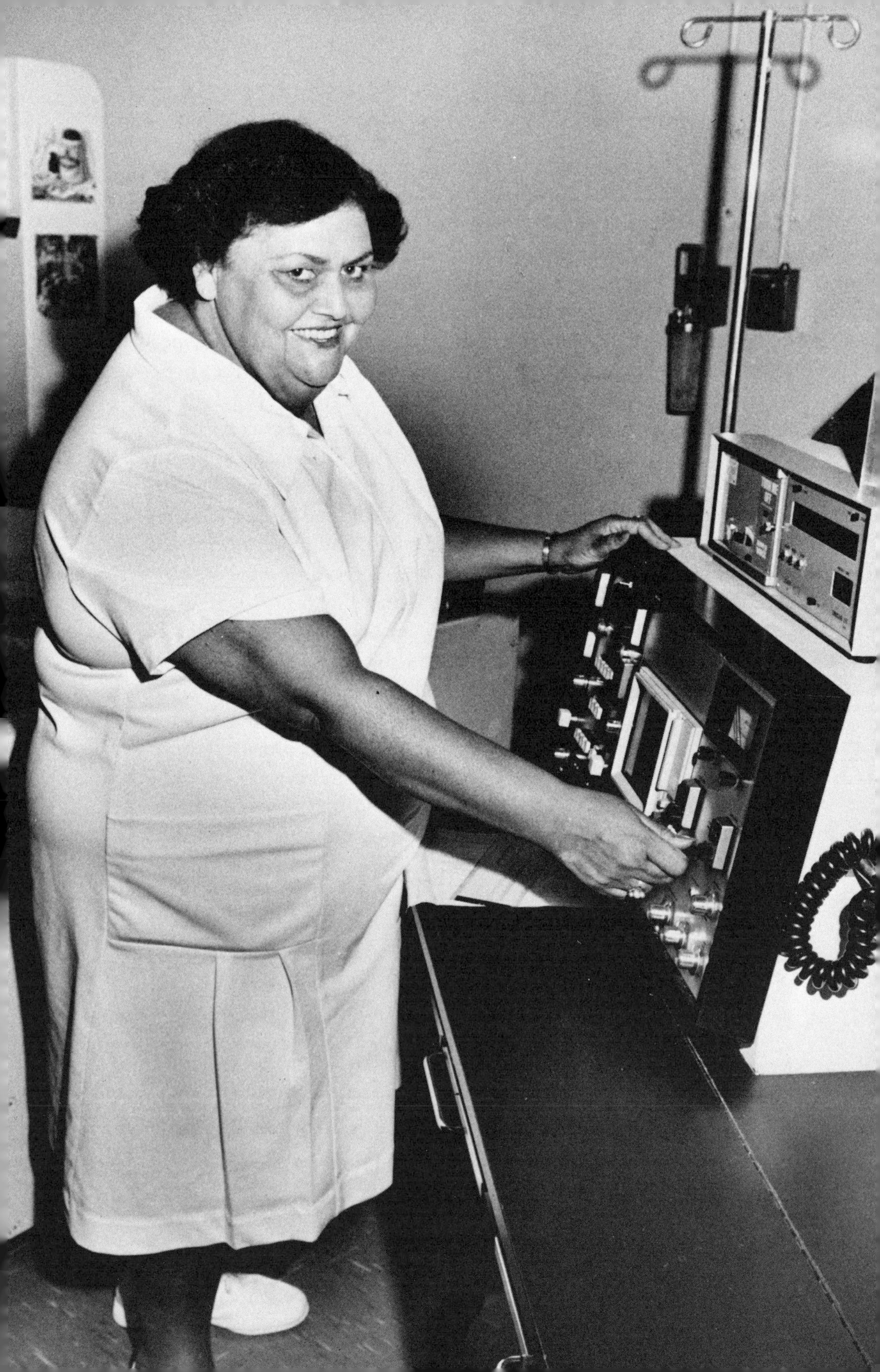

happiest at the bedside. Most people who go into nursing want to serve other people. You don't serve by shuffling papers at a desk! We ought to have three-year programs for people who want to work at the bedside, with additional years for people who want to go into administration and education."

Each state has a Nurse Practice Act which lists the duties nurses can legally perform in the course of their work. Someone once said that if these laws were all rigidly enforced, patients in hospitals would never get any treatment. The situation, however, is not quite as extreme as that. The New York State Act defines nursing in part as "diagnosing and treating human responses to actual or potential health problems through such services as case-finding, health counseling, and provision of care supportive to or restorative of life and well-being, and executing medical regimens prescribed by a licensed or otherwise legally authorized physician or dentist."

Many nurses today want these regulations to have more specific language. These women are proponents of a concept that has arisen since the advent of the women's movement, that of an extended or expanded role for nurses. They are trying to eliminate the "handmaiden" image of previous years, whereby nurses were seen as women who were there simply to carry out physicians' orders. Instead, they want an explicit statement of their special responsibility in providing health care. They admit that this responsibility overlaps with that of the doctor to some extent, but claim that it also commands an area independent of his domain, an area where their first duty is not to him, but to their patients.

The expanded-role concept has been implemented in the

Like every other field, medicine needs its administrators. This nurse is in charge of the radiology department at a large hospital.

past ten years or so by the development of a number of new professional opportunities for nurses. One is that of the nurse-practitioner. This is a nurse who can go into private practice —opening an office, hanging out a shingle, receiving visits, making house calls, and referring patients to a doctor when that is necessary. Actually, this kind of work is not as much an innovation as it might seem. Nurses have practiced on their own in poor and underserved areas for many years. When the Frontier Nursing Service was founded in 1925, the nurses it sent out into rural and sparsely populated areas of the country set up clinics, giving the people there the first professional health care they had ever had. Also, nurses in the Public Health and Visiting Nurse Services of big cities have always had to use great sensitivity, responsibility, and initiative in dealing with the needs of their patients, who usually live in the poorest, unhealthiest, and most crime-ridden urban areas.

Nurse-practitioners can also work in schools, outpatient clinics, and group practices, where, among other things, they can serve as a telephone front line. In such a situation, the patient calling up with a complaint talks not to an office receptionist with an appointment book, but to a health professional trained to get a history, give preliminary counseling, and make an educated decision as to what care the patient will need. As a colleague, not an employee, of the physicians with whom she works, the nurse-practitioner can then explain to them what appears to be needed, even if it means a change in scheduling, thus acting as the patient's advocate. By seeing the patient through the various specialists he or she may encounter, and by providing instruction about home care, she can become a source of remedy for the fragmentation many people believe is developing between the various medical specialties.

A number of training hospitals give courses to equip licensed R.N.'s to assume this role. One, the PRIMEX program, was set up at New York Hospital-Cornell Medical School in 1971. It lasts one year, including 4½ months of classwork and 7½ months of clinical internship.

Nurse-clinicians are expanded-role nurses who work in the intensive care units of hospitals. They must understand the sophisticated equipment in use there and know all the possible side effects of the drugs given their critically ill patients. Some nurse-clinicians come from masters' programs in clinical specialties. Others are diploma nurses who have taken a special 1–1½ year training course.

Nurse-midwives are a major component of the expanded-role corps—there are about 1,200 of them delivering babies in the United States today. Sixteen medical schools currently give courses in nurse-midwifery. To enter these programs you must be a diploma or baccalaureate-trained nurse with a year's experience in obstetrical work. After a two-year course of study, including such courses as embryology and reproductive anatomy, and clinical experience including attendance at a certain number of deliveries, you will be eligible to take the certifying examination given by the American College of Nurse-Midwives. Certified nurse-midwives are allowed to manage normal deliveries (ones not requiring a forceps or a Caesarian section) in most states, although the laws in this area are constantly changing.

Nurses involved in the drive to institute the expanded-role concept emphasize that they are not trying to become doctors. They say that they are merely trying to become nurses in the most fully realized sense of the word. What do doctors say with regard to this issue?

Most doctors express great respect for and dependence upon the nurses with whom they work. One said he would be more inclined to trust the judgment of a good operating room nurse with years of experience behind her than he would that of a first-year resident. The days when house physicians summoned nurses like cocker spaniels by snapping their fingers are almost a thing of the past. However, many nurses still feel that male doctors are unable to regard nurses as either true colleagues or equals. Something called the "doctor-nurse game" can result from this inability. This is a game in which a nurse makes a suggestion but does so very, very carefully, so that the doctor will not feel that she is trying to tell him how to do his job. "Male physicians do not like to be criticized by females," one doctor remarked about this problem, "but the nurse can spot things the doctor can't, and I for one don't feel it makes for bad patient care to have the nurse question the physician." The responsibility for "spotting" everything about her patients' conditions and for reporting anything dangerous at once is in fact one of the most important aspects of a nurse's job. Still, some physicians are afraid that in their quest for professional prestige nurses will abuse this charge, taking on more responsibility than their training warrants.

Most nurses feel this alarm is uncalled for. "The State Education Board, which writes the Nurse Practice Act, is right to be concerned about patients," one nurses training school officer said. "But the AMA wants to add language to those acts which goes beyond our ability to police our own profession. This is unreasonable. *We* don't tell *them* how to practice."

Most nurses consider the new concept of the physician's assistant to be the most obvious and serious effort on the part of the medical profession to halt the expanded-role movement. Begun in 1966, when the first physician's assistant training program was set up at Duke University, the P.A. idea was originally an attempt to integrate military medical corpsmen (medics) returning from the war in Vietnam into the civilian health-care structure. There are now many such training programs around the country, most of them two years in length of study, usually incorporating nine months of basic science and fifteen months of clinical experience. Some require college work—although not necessarily a degree—in addition to a high school diploma. You can get a list of these training programs and other data from the Association of Physician's Assistant Programs, 2120 L Street, NW, The Gelman Building, Suite 210, Washington, D.C., 20037. The examination for certification as a physician's assistant is administered by the AMA's Council on Medical Education. By law, P.A.s work under the supervision of doctors, who are responsible for their performance. They can take medical histories, do routine lab work such as blood and urine tests, remove casts and stitches, accompany doctors on rounds, and transcribe and carry out orders. Most doctors are extremely busy people, and the services provided by these trained paraprofessionals can be very valuable.

"But," nurses say, "we were here all the time, willing and able to do all that—and more. We have more training than the P.A.s. Why not use us? Why make up a whole new category?" Many nurses are bitter about the way the AMA came out for the P.A. idea at exactly the same time the expanded-role movement was getting off the ground. They view it as a deliberate effort on the part of the medical profession to erect a male block (most P.A.s are young men) against the nurses' new professional aspirations. (An added reason for nurses' resentment could well be financial. A P.A. with two years of technical training can expect to make $10–15,000 a year, whereas a hospital R.N. probably cannot hope to go above $12,000. Some operating room nurses may get $15,000. Male nurses, who make up 2 percent of the profession, are often able to get slightly higher salaries, but they would still have trouble supporting a family on their earnings, and it has been suggested that this is one reason why so few men enter the profession. There are others, of course, primarily having to do with the image of nursing as a profession for women.)

In spite of all this, however, frustrated activist nurses still reserve their chief anger not for P.A.s or their sponsoring physicians, or the AMA, or male hospital administrators, or the lawmakers, but for other nurses—the great number of them who simply do not want to alter their role as the passively nurturing handmaiden. Because most nurses choose their profession out of a desire to help people; because their training frequently takes place in rigidly structured, sexually segregated surroundings; because nurses can be penalized if they speak up when they see something being done incorrectly or improperly; because many nurses are personally conservative women who do not want to do anything that may cause them to be identified with the "bra burners"—for all these reasons, most nurses neither want nor are willing to take action to change the way their role is expressed. This is not to say that they are not proud of their profession. They are talented, hardworking women, without whom health care in this country would be a fleshless, nerveless skeleton. Still, these women are a thorn in the sides of some of their sisters.

"Nurses are their own worst enemies," declares one woman physician. "They should be getting better nurse practice acts. They should be working for collective bargaining and grievance procedures. Instead, they're content to let male hospital administrators tell them what to do. They could be doing much more." Time and again, nurses interested in securing such goals as those discussed above have quit in angry despair over the persistent refusal of their co-workers to assume leadership and responsibility. Regretfully, they cite the fact that most nurses are not interested in organizing—only 25 percent are members of the ANA.

There may be another reason for the difficulty in finding a workable political power base in the nursing profession: the high turnover rate, which one statistician put at 60 percent a year. Perhaps the chief reason so many women leave nursing is that they need time for their families. Ironically, even though nursing is seen as a woman's profession almost by definition, it is actually less amenable to the demands of a home and family than medicine. Doctors (as you will see in the next chapter) can arrange to work part-time, or half days, or only until three p.m., but most nurses do not have this option. They must put in a full forty-hour week if they work in a hospital or a doctor's office, and although many women physicians put in long hours too, nurses are often less willing to take that kind of time away from their families. So, while in many respects it is a natural arena for the newest struggles of feminism, the nursing profession may well not be the scene of an overall revolution in the near future—although some women pin their hopes for change on the infusion of fresh, young blood. "The only way we can start accomplishing things," one of them said, "is to encourage more bright young women to come into the profession. Then maybe they can start going out and putting into practice the idea of all we can do, and when that happens everyone will gain—the overworked doctors in private offices, the generations of nurses yet to come, and most of all—and most importantly of all—the patients."

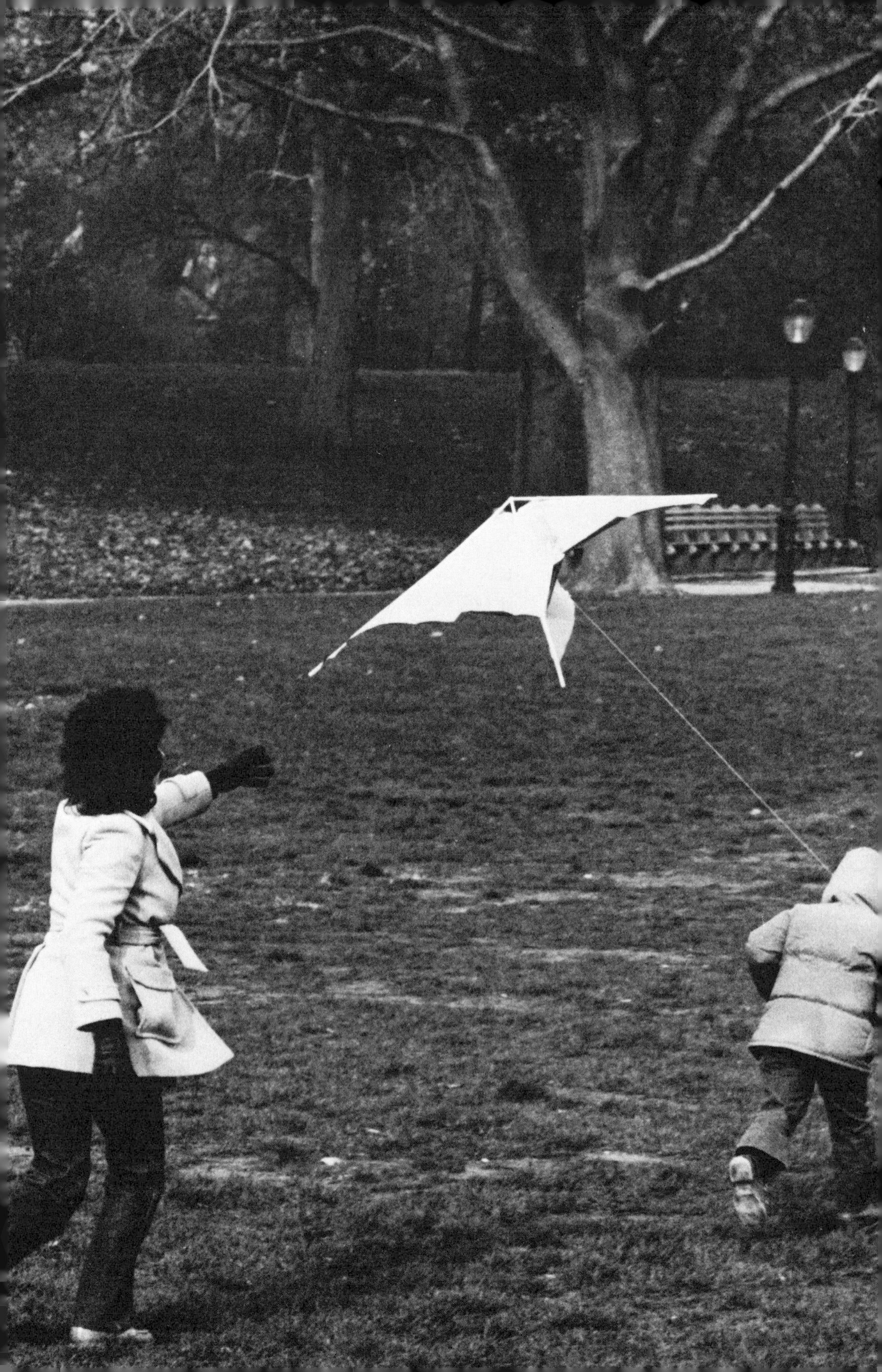

10

Combining a Practice With a Family

Women have compared the combining of medical practice with family life to walking a tightrope over a gorge, or juggling sixteen oranges. You must realize that you can't maintain two full-time jobs, they warn. Some say you shouldn't even try. One nurse, asked what she thought of women physicians, answered, "I'm concerned about their families. If you're going to pursue a medical career, maybe it's even better not to have children. I know a lot of people would jump up and down at that, but I really don't approve of having someone else bring up your children." And a doctor, who was worrying not about her colleagues' children, but about their professional dedication, arrived at almost the same point from the opposite direction: "Young women would consider this old-fashioned or brainwashed, but you have to give medicine a priority. You've had all that training and you should make yourself good. You can marry and have children of course, but if you're not a good doctor first, then no one will respect you."

And yet women are succeeding in both spheres every day, in clinics, hospitals, and private offices all over the country, so don't let anyone tell you that you can't do it too.

The overwhelming majority of women physicians who were interviewed for this book were married, and most had two or more children. Indeed, statistics show that women who go into medicine are not only as likely to marry as women in the general population (though they tend to do so a little later), but are likely to have slightly *larger* families than other professional women. In addition, they are less likely than other women to change their professional patterns (hours, etc.) once they have children. Nevertheless, many women still feel there must be a contradiction in this scheme somewhere. Jessica had an experience which bears this out. "I had given a two-hour seminar in embryology at Cornell," she remembered, "and at the end of it every woman in the hall came up to me and asked me how old I was and how many children I had. They were absolutely the last questions I'd expected! I learned a lot that day. When another woman lets her hair down with you, you can see what's really bothering her."

Women are not the only ones who are bothered by the question. A lot of men in the profession have long worried that women are a poor medical school admissions risk because they do things like get married and have babies, which causes them to stop working, which means that the cost of their whole medical education was a waste. Fortunately, not all are as nasty (or as mistaken) as the cardiologist who told his class on the first day of school, "It will be interesting to go to your fiftieth reunion and see how many of the women in this room have ever done a full day's work." But there are many who agree with the admissions officer who said, somewhat more temperately, "This year I had to insist we take only the above-average women," because he thought there was too much risk of their not spending enough time actually practicing to make educating them worthwhile.

It *is* true that women physicians who are single publish more, that they belong to more medical societies, and attend more conferences than those who are married. It is also true that when a woman doctor has a family, the number of hours she works is in inverse proportion to the number of children she has. But it is *not* true that most women doctors simply take off when their first child is born and are never seen or heard from again. The vast majority goes back to work soon after their babies are born; only a minority stays home for a year or two thereafter. (This practice was more common in the past than it is today.) But the woman who leaves practice for maternity and then stays away for years is practically unheard of.

So how do they manage?

Part of the answer, though only part, lies in the fact that a medical career no longer means being the only G.P. for fifty miles (or even blocks) around, nor does it mean having to be on call night and day for any and all emergencies. Whether we like it or not, medicine in this country just is not practiced that way any more. For one thing, more and more doctors are going into the specialized areas of medicine, many of which afford the possibility of more regular hours. Organ specialties, like ophthalmology (eye), otolaryngology (ear, nose, and throat), and dermatology (skin) generally have little emergency or night work. Physicians in the service specialties, so called because they render services to other doctors—anesthesiology, radiology (X rays), and pathology—are employed by institutions and typically work on a fixed schedule.

In addition, even for the physician in a primary care specialty such as family practice or pediatrics, there is the possibility of group practice, in which she can have set work hours. The woman going into medicine today has, in fact, an almost unlimited choice of jobs that will take up only as much of her time as she chooses. She can work three days or four days or five mornings a week in a hospital clinic. She can be a school doctor and get off every day at three. She can have a nine-to-five job in public health or occupational medicine. More than one woman physician has remarked that medicine is one of the *best* fields for a woman who wants both a career and a family, precisely because of the wealth of options it offers.

There are also a number of ways in which life has been made

easier for women during their training. One is the NIRMP's plan for married or engaged medical students who want to be together during their internships. You and your fiance or husband can fill out a special internship application requesting that you both be placed in the same program, hospital, or community. You will be placed in the hospital highest on your list that chooses you both. You can also specify that if placement together is impossible, you want one of you to be placed at his or her highest possible choice, while the other is left unplaced—it will be up to the two of you to decide which partner will be the one so placed.

There are part-time internship and residency programs offered to women with children. One of the best-known of these is the one in psychiatry at Flower Fifth Avenue Hospital in New York City, established in 1962. It lasts four years instead of three, with participants working nine to five and having evenings, weekends, and school vacations off. They get the same salary overall that full-time residents get for their more concentrated three years. A number of hospitals around the country have instituted similar programs. Nevertheless, the number of women who go into these programs is small. Many believe there is something second-class about a part-time arrangement, and one said tartly, "The best way to get women discriminated against is to offer them the 'privilege' of a watered-down program. Such efforts cannot help but result in dissatisfaction among male house officers, and poor training for the woman who feels like a fifth wheel." "At times there is resentment by the men," one male physician in a hospital with such a program agreed, "but as they get to know the women personally, this lessens. The men need time off too, to help if their wives are sick, for example, and they get it without any difficulty." A more difficult situation arises when the hospital has not announced an official policy about part-time work, but simply lets it be known that it will make an ad hoc arrangement if a woman requests it. Each woman involved may indeed feel she is asking for special favors on the basis of her sex—a position she is understandably eager to avoid.

With or without the aid of such part-time arrangements, a little over one-third of all medical women do have their first children at some point in their training, according to Carol Lopate in *Woman in Medicine.* Some do it while still in medical school, and they usually find it to be extremely difficult. Some believe that this practice may be one of the factors contributing to the higher dropout rate of women medical students. Of course, it does not always work out badly; one woman who became pregnant in her sophomore year admitted she had not intended to, and that it made for a great many problems, but now she is glad that she did. "If I had waited until my residency was over to have a baby, my oldest son would be nine now instead of sixteen," she said. "You don't want to start folding diapers just when you've finally finished your training." Some women have become pregnant and given birth during their internships, although such a situation is especially demanding. Most women who have babies during their training do so during their residencies, which may be the least hectic period, even if you are not on a part-time schedule. One woman who was nursing her baby simply took him along on her rounds in a sling, stepping into an empty room when mealtime approached. Another had her husband bring their son to the hospital "for supper" when she was on night call.

But all these considerations—part-time study, part-time clinic work where you can write your own ticket, hospital work where someone may be able to cover for you, group work where someone *will* cover for you—are only half the story. The other half, of course, is that you are going to have to have someone taking care of your children at least part of the time.

That sounds so obvious that one would think everyone would have figured it out long ago, and then come to a decision as to what to do about it. A few years ago, however, when the Medical Women's International Association sent out a questionnaire to its members which included one query about household help, it was astonished at the volume of the response. A veritable avalanche of letters poured in, saying, "Yes! Household help is a problem, all right! Yes! It's hard to get! Yes! I could have worked more if only I'd had more help. HELP!" Commenting on this in an article in *The Woman Physician,* Dr. Matilda Vaschak said, "Household help is, in my opinion, a woman physician's greatest problem. All the rest are miniscule by comparison."

So how do they do it? Quite a few were helped out by their mothers or mothers-in-law. One cardiologist in private practice opened her first office in a two-family house with her husband's parents living in the upper story, and that solved the problem for her. A pediatrician in public health said she could not have succeeded without her mother-in-law—even though she had a housekeeper—because the housekeeper didn't always show up. One remark that kept cropping up about these helping grandmothers is that they are unfailingly reliable; they would never let a grandchild down. Whereas hired help is not so dependable. As one woman pointed out, "If the surgeon cuts at eight a.m., and your housekeeper hasn't shown up by 7:30 . . . !" And another woman said, "I was lucky that my mother was living in the same city when my boy was young, because I just wasn't interested in having anyone else take care of him." Not everyone feels that way, however, and it is interesting to note that most of the women who asked their mothers for help were in their forties or older. This may indicate that young women today are less willing to have their mothers watch their children. Or it may simply reflect the fact that the mothers of today's young professional women are somewhat more likely to be working themselves, and simply cannot take the time.

For most women, then, help must be hired. This usually means placing ads and interviewing people, which can be an intimidating process for someone who has never done it before and who is not sure what to ask. Another thing about hiring people is that you sometimes have to fire them too. A number of mothers lamented that they had never been able to keep anyone longer than two years. Most women consider it a plus if a housekeeper can stay long enough to know everyone well, and in time become almost like a member of the family. Those who consider themselves luckiest of all, and who are least likely to talk about child-care as a serious problem, are those who have had just one helper all the way through.

Getting good, dependable help is one of the greatest problems, but whether someone is referred by friends, or whether you have to rely on personnel agencies, you will still make out. Even though the problems of getting help may reduce your work hours temporarily, I did not talk to one woman who allowed her career to come to a full stop because of that difficulty. All those who had decided they wanted to work, did so somehow. Those who stopped working did so for a different reason: they wanted more time with their children.

"I never was willing to sacrifice raising my children—not until they were three, certainly," said one. "They say that the quality of the time you spend with your children is more important than the quantity, but you have to invest a certain amount of time with your kids just to know them and watch them develop." One pediatrician interrupted her graduate work (and, significantly, she does not say "I dropped out" or "I quit," but rather, "I took a year off") between her residency and fellowship to get married and have a baby, and she recommends it. "It's very important to learn how to be a mother, and there's nothing like trying it. I wouldn't have been able to do it again for the next three years." These women are not apologetic about the time they took from their work to give to their children; they are happy that they did what they thought was right.

Should you follow their example? Some women say yes, definitely. One psychiatrist invoked the findings of her discipline, saying, "Psychological tests show that for a child to learn to trust and relate well, he should be brought up with a constant, close relationship. I was a psychiatrist exclusively when my daughter was little, and she has said that she felt then that she wasn't very important to me. I regret that I didn't stay home with her more."

In the end, of course, it will be up to you. Some women decide not to stay home precisely because they feel it would have been worse for their families if they had, and not better. One dentist remembered, "I worked three days a week after my daughter was born and I went crazy. She was happier when I went back to five days—that way I had more patience. I just can't be home. I worked until ten days before she was born—people used to jump out of the chair when they saw me coming. I told my husband before we were married: 'If you want to marry me, that's the way it's going to be.' "

That last sentence, by the way, deserves your special attention. There is no subject on which women physicians are more unanimous than the need for a sympathetic, encouraging, understanding husband. Practically every woman who has ever spoken or written about her career mentions it, whether asked to or not! "My husband was terrifically supportive." "Your husband has to respect your commitment to your career. He has to be able to accept the fact that you may make more money than he does." "He always let me know he was behind me 100 percent. That's been the biggest single factor in making my career a success." When I had heard so many of these comments that I felt prompted to remark on them, the doctor I was talking to said, "That's probably because a woman with the confidence and ambition to want a medical career in the first place would probably not be drawn to a man who was reluctant to support her goals."

If you do decide to take some time off for your family, you should know about the retraining programs some medical schools have set up to help women readjust to their professional duties. Such programs are necessary because so many new things are constantly being learned about medicine, that doctors are of necessity students all their lives. Keeping up with these advances is as much a part of a conscientious physician's professional responsibility as is taking care of her patients. Losing touch with the profession even for a short while can mean falling considerably behind: one cardiologist estimated that a doctor has to go to a minimum of three conferences a year just to keep up. And it is such things as conferences and journal reading that are often the first things to go when a woman physician begins to feel the crunch, even if she keeps on working. Consequently a woman returning to practice after a period away may feel she is at an intimidating disadvantage.

The Women's Medical College of Pennsylvania has set up a nine-month retraining course for women who live near enough to commute to the college. There is a special six-week session for those who have to come in and find room and board. The Presbyterian Hospital Medical Center in San Francisco also has a program, set up in 1966, for women who are already board-eligible; others are offered a rotation through specialties. Not everyone considers these programs a good idea, or at least they didn't once. The sociologist Alice Rossi worried about the implications thus: "There is a danger that by institutionalizing the withdrawal-and-return pattern of college-educated women, we may reduce even further the likelihood that women will enter the top professions." But Rossi was writing over ten years ago, when the idea of women being full-time professionals was not quite so firmly established as it is today. People were still remembering the feminine mystique of the fifties, when popular opinion did not expect mothers to have full-time careers, even if they were highly educated.

Today, with more women working at all levels than ever before, and—more importantly—with more people understanding that they will do so and believing that they should, I am certain that no woman will hesitate to stake her claim for the best of both possible worlds, no matter how she decides to go about it.

Appendix

MEDICAL SCHOOLS IN THE UNITED STATES AND CANADA

United States

Alabama
University of Alabama School of Medicine *
University of South Alabama College of Medicine *

Arizona
University of Arizona College of Medicine *

Arkansas
University of Arkansas School of Medicine *

California
University of California, Davis, School of Medicine *
University of California, Irvine, California College of Medicine *
University of California, Los Angeles (UCLA), School of Medicine *
University of California, San Diego, School of Medicine *
University of California, San Francisco, School of Medicine *
Loma Linda University School of Medicine
University of Southern California School of Medicine
Stanford University School of Medicine

Colorado
University of Colorado School of Medicine *

* Publicly supported schools.

Connecticut
University of Connecticut School of Medicine *
Yale University School of Medicine

District of Columbia
Georgetown University School of Medicine
George Washington University School of Medicine and Health Sciences
Howard University College of Medicine

Florida
University of Florida College of Medicine *
University of Miami School of Medicine
University of South Florida College of Medicine *

Georgia
Emory University School of Medicine
Medical College of Georgia School of Medicine *

Hawaii
University of Hawaii School of Medicine *

Illinois
University of Health Sciences, The Chicago Medical School
University of Chicago Pritzker School of Medicine
University of Illinois College of Medicine *
Loyola University of Chicago Stritch School of Medicine
Northwestern University Medical School
Rush Medical College of Rush University
Southern Illinois University School of Medicine *

Indiana
Indiana University School of Medicine *

Iowa
University of Iowa College of Medicine *

Kansas
University of Kansas School of Medicine *

Kentucky
University of Kentucky College of Medicine *
University of Louisville School of Medicine *

Louisiana
Louisiana State University School of Medicine in New Orleans *
Louisiana State University School of Medicine in Shreveport *
Tulane University School of Medicine

Maryland
Johns Hopkins University School of Medicine
University of Maryland School of Medicine *

Massachusetts
Boston University School of Medicine

Michigan
Michigan State University College of Human Medicine *
University of Michigan Medical School *
Wayne State University School of Medicine *

Minnesota
University of Minnesota—Duluth School of Medicine
University of Minnesota Medical School—Minneapolis *

Mississippi
University of Mississippi School of Medicine *

Missouri
University of Missouri—Columbia School of Medicine *
University of Missouri—Kansas City School of Medicine *
St. Louis University School of Medicine
Washington University School of Medicine

Nebraska
Creighton University School of Medicine
University of Nebraska College of Medicine *

Nevada
University of Nevada, Reno, School of Medical Sciences *

New Hampshire
Dartmouth Medical School

New Jersey
College of Medicine and Dentistry of New Jersey, New Jersey Medical School *
College of Medicine and Dentistry of New Jersey, Rutgers Medical School *

New Mexico
University of New Mexico School of Medicine *

New York
Albany Medical College of Union University
Albert Einstein College of Medicine of Yeshiva University
Columbia University College of Physicians and Surgeons
Cornell University Medical College
Mount Sinai School of Medicine of the City University of New York
New York Medical College
New York University School of Medicine
University of Rochester School of Medicine and Dentistry
State University of New York at Buffalo School of Medicine *
State University of New York Downstate Medical Center College of Medicine *
State University of New York at Stony Brook Health Sciences Center School of Medicine *
State University of New York Upstate Medical Center College of Medicine *

North Carolina
Bowman Gray School of Medicine of Wake Forest University
Duke University School of Medicine
University of North Carolina School of Medicine *

North Dakota
University of North Dakota School of Medicine *

Ohio
Case Western Reserve University School of Medicine
University of Cincinnati College of Medicine *
Medical College of Ohio at Toledo *
Ohio State University College of Medicine *
Wright State University School of Medicine *

Oklahoma
University of Oklahoma College of Medicine *

Oregon
University of Oregon Medical School *

Pennsylvania
Hahnemann Medical College of Philadelphia
Jefferson Medical College of Thomas Jefferson University
Medical College of Pennsylvania
Pennsylvania State University College of Medicine *
University of Pennsylvania School of Medicine
University of Pittsburgh School of Medicine *
Temple University School of Medicine *

Rhode Island
Brown University Program in Medicine

South Carolina
Medical University of South Carolina College of Medicine *

South Dakota
University of South Dakota School of Medicine *

Tennessee
Meharry Medical College School of Medicine
University of Tennessee College of Medicine *
Vanderbilt University School of Medicine *

Texas
Baylor College of Medicine
Texas Tech University School of Medicine *
University of Texas Health Science Center at Dallas Southwestern Medical School *
University of Texas Medical Branch at Galveston School of Medicine *
University of Texas Medical School at Houston *
University of Texas Health Science Center at San Antonio Medical School *

Utah
University of Utah College of Medicine *

Vermont
University of Vermont College of Medicine *

Virginia
Eastern Virginia Medical School *
Medical College of Virginia School of Medicine of Virginia Commonwealth University *
University of Virginia School of Medicine *

Washington
University of Washington School of Medicine *

West Virginia
West Virginia University School of Medicine *

Wisconsin
Medical College of Wisconsin
University of Wisconsin Medical School *

Canada

Alberta
University of Alberta, Faculty of Medicine
University of Calgary, Faculty of Medicine

British Columbia
University of British Columbia, Faculty of Medicine

Manitoba
University of Manitoba, Faculty of Medicine

Newfoundland
Memorial University of Newfoundland, Medical School

Nova Scotia
Dalhousie University, Faculty of Medicine

Ontario
McMaster University, School of Medicine
University of Ottawa, Faculty of Medicine
Queen's University, Faculty of Medicine
University of Toronto, Faculty of Medicine
University of Western Ontario, Faculty of Medicine

Quebec
Laval University, Faculty of Medicine
McGill University, Faculty of Medicine
University of Montreal, Faculty of Medicine
University of Sherbrooke, Faculty of Medicine

Saskatchewan
University of Saskatchewan, College of Medicine

Bibliography

Campbell, Margaret A., M.D. *Why Would a Girl Go into Medicine? Medical Education in the United States: A Guide for Women.* The Feminist Press, Old Westbury, New York, 1973.

Career Choices for Women in Medicine. The American Medical Women's Association, 1973.

Directory of Approved Internships and Residencies, 1973–74. The American Medical Association, 1973.

Edelson, Edward. "The Women Doctors," three part series in *The New York Daily News,* April 19–21, 1975.

Ingelfinger, Franz. "Doctor-Women," *New England Journal of Medicine,* Vol. 291, 1974, pp. 303–304.

Jacobson, Beverly, and Wendy Jacobson. "Only 8%: A Look at Women in Medicine," *Civil Rights Digest,* Summer 1975.

Jolly, H. P. "Women Physicians on U.S. Medical School Faculties," *Journal of Medical Education,* Vol. 50, Aug. 1975, pp. 825–828.

Jussum, Judith, and Charlotte Muller. "Medical Education for Women: How Good an Investment?" *Journal of Medical Education,* Vol. 50, June 1975, pp. 571–579.

Lopate, Carol. *Women in Medicine.* Johns Hopkins Press, Baltimore, 1968.

"Malpractice Crisis: How It's Hurting Medical Care," *U.S. News and World Report,* Vol. 78, May 26, 1975, pp. 32–34.

"Malpractice Crunch," *Science News,* Vol. 103, May 26, 1973, pp. 338–339.

Maselka, Ronald J. *N.I.H.—A Profile,* 14-article series in *The Buffalo Evening News,* reprinted as Department of Health, Education and Welfare publication No. 74-21.

Nemir, Rosa, M.D. "Women Doctors and Others," *Journal of the American Medical Women's Association,* Vol. 28, Sept. 1973, pp. 475–477.

Silver, George A. "Women in Medicine," editorial in *The Nation,* Vol. 220, June 21, 1975, p. 741.

Spiro, Howard E. "Myths and Mirths: Women in Medicine," *New England Journal of Medicine,* Vol. 292, 1975, pp. 354–356.

Tabershaw, I. R. "Whose 'Agent' Is the Occupational Physician?" *Archives of Environmental Health,* Vol. 30, Aug. 1975, pp. 412–416.

Vaschak, Matilda, M.D. "Household Help: The Woman Doctor's Gordian Knot," *The Woman Physician,* Vol. 25, 1970.

Wadler, Joyce. "Woman of the Week: Dr. Nina Lief," *New York Post,* April 24, 1976.

For Further Reading

Campbell, Margaret A., M.D. *Why Would a Girl Go into Medicine? Medical Education in the United States: A Guide for Women.* The Feminist Press, Old Westbury, New York, 1973. A book about sexism in medical school, consisting mostly of respondents' answers to a questionnaire sent out by the author.

Directory of Approved Internships and Residencies, published annually by the American Medical Association. A huge paperback volume which, in addition to listing all the approved graduate programs in the country, provides dozens of graphs and charts showing the distribution of foreign medical students, women, minorities, and other groups throughout the specialties, as well as the different types of graduate training. Wonderful if statistics fascinate you. You can order it from the Order Department, OP-378, American Medical Association, 535 North Dearborn Street, Chicago, Illinois, 60610.

Fenten, D. X. *Ms.—M.D.* Westminster Press, Philadelphia, 1973. A book about medical training for the young woman considering medicine as a career. Contains a list of all American medical schools and their entrance requirements.

Lopate, Carol. *Women in Medicine,* Johns Hopkins Press, Baltimore, 1968. Chapters on the approach to medical school, from high school through college: training, graduate work and practice. A solid, fact-filled book, although some of the comments have become a little dated.

Index

About the Author

A graduate of Barnard College, Carol Jochnowitz has written a number of books and articles on medical topics. The current project grew from her interest in the women's movement, combined with a lifelong fascination with the medical profession. She lives with her husband and two daughters in New York City, where she was born. *Careers in Medicine for the New Woman* is her first book for young adult readers.